P9-BZZ-469

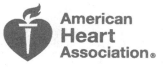

American
Heart
Association®

Healthy Fats,
Low-Cholesterol
Cookbook

FIFTH EDITION

also by the
American Heart Association

....

American Heart Association Grill It, Braise It, Broil It

American Heart Association Go Fresh

American Heart Association The Go Red For Women Cookbook

American Heart Association Eat Less Salt

American Heart Association Healthy Slow Cooker Cookbook

American Heart Association Complete Guide to Women's Heart Health

American Heart Association Healthy Family Meals

American Heart Association No-Fad Diet, 2nd Edition

The New American Heart Association Cookbook, 8th Edition

American Heart Association Low-Salt Cookbook, 4th Edition

American Heart Association Quick & Easy Meals

American Heart Association Quick & Easy Cookbook, 2nd Edition

American Heart Association Meals in Minutes

American Heart Association One-Dish Meals

American Heart Association Low-Calorie Cookbook

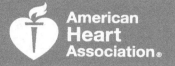

American Heart Association®

healthy fats, low-cholesterol cookbook

FIFTH EDITION

delicious recipes to help reduce bad fats and lower your cholesterol

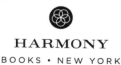

HARMONY

BOOKS · NEW YORK

Copyright © 2015 by American Heart Association

All rights reserved.

Published in the United States by Harmony Books, an
imprint of the Crown Publishing Group, a division of
Penguin Random House LLC, New York.

www.crownpublishing.com

Harmony Books is a registered trademark and the Circle
colophon is a trademark of Penguin Random House LLC.

Previous editions published in the United States
by Clarkson Potter/Publishers, an imprint of
the Crown Publishing Group, a division of
Penguin Random House LLC, New York,
in 1989, 1997, 2004, and 2008.

Your contribution to the American Heart Association
supports research that helps make publications like this
possible. For more information, call 1-800-AHA-USA1
(1-800-242-8721) or contact us online at
www.americanheart.org.

LIBRARY OF CONGRESS
CATALOGING-IN-PUBLICATION DATA
is available upon request.

ISBN 978-0-553-44716-3
eBook ISBN 978-0-553-44717-0

Printed in the United States of America

Book design by Barbara M. Bachman
Cover design by Gabriel Levine
Cover photograph by Lucy Schaeffer

10 9 8 7 6 5 4 3 2 1

FIFTH EDITION

contents

ACKNOWLEDGMENTS   vii

PREFACE   ix

FATS, CHOLESTEROL, AND HEART HEALTH   1

HEALTHY FOOD, HEALTHY HEART   5

HEALTHY LIFESTYLE, HEALTHY HEART   19

recipes

Appetizers, Snacks, and Beverages   29

Soups   51

Salads and Salad Dressings   71

Seafood   103

Poultry   141

Meats   179

Vegetarian Entrées   211

Vegetables and Side Dishes   247

Breads and Breakfast Dishes   277

Desserts   293

appendixes

APPENDIX A. HEALTHY SHOPPING STRATEGIES   319

APPENDIX B. HEALTHY COOKING STRATEGIES   325

APPENDIX C. HEALTHY DINING OUT STRATEGIES   339

APPENDIX D. THE SCIENCE BEHIND THE RECOMMENDATIONS   343

APPENDIX E. RISK FACTORS FOR HEART DISEASE AND STROKE   346

APPENDIX F. WARNING SIGNS FOR HEART ATTACK AND STROKE   349

INDEX   351

acknowledgments

AMERICAN HEART ASSOCIATION
CONSUMER PUBLICATIONS

Acting Director: Deborah A. Renza
Senior Editor: Robin P. Loveman
Assistant Managing Editor: Roberta W. Sullivan

RECIPE DEVELOPERS FOR FIFTH EDITION

Ellen Boeke
Barbara Seelig Brown
Meredith Deeds
Nancy S. Hughes
Annie King
Jackie Mills, M.S., R.D.
Kathryn Moore
Carol Ritchie
Julie Shapero, R.D., L.D.
Roxanne Wyss

RECIPE DEVELOPERS FOR PREVIOUS EDITIONS

Sherry Ferguson
Nancy S. Hughes
Annie King
Laureen Mody, R.D.
Leni Reed, R.D.
Carol Ritchie
Julie Shapero, R.D., L.D.
Linda Foley Woodrum

NUTRITION ANALYST

Tammi Hancock, R.D.

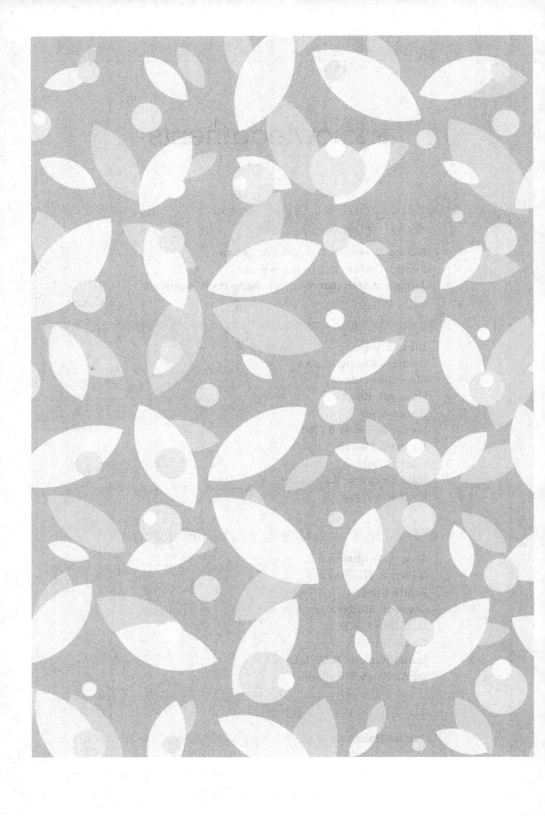

preface

At the American Heart Association, we know that managing what you eat is one of the best ways to take care of your heart. Following the updated American Heart Association dietary and lifestyle recommendations, this revised edition of the *American Heart Association Healthy Fats, Low-Cholesterol Cookbook* is a reliable, science-based resource for nutritious and delicious recipes as well as practical advice on how to achieve good heart health.

The *American Heart Association Healthy Fats, Low-Cholesterol Cookbook, Fifth Edition,* will guide you to make healthy food choices every day to help you control your cholesterol level and enjoy an overall heart-healthy diet. The 200 tasty recipes—including 50 new ones—show how you can savor the great flavor of food while limiting your intake of unhealthy fats. Replacing saturated and trans fats with better-for-you fats (monounsaturated and polyunsaturated) can help lower the concentration of low-density lipoprotein (LDL) cholesterol in your blood, which will help lower your risk factor for heart disease and stroke.

In addition to new recipes in every chapter, this cookbook offers easy-to-use strategies for healthier shopping, cooking, and dining out; information on what types of foods to include and limit in your diet; and overall healthy lifestyle recommendations. As the nation's most trusted authority on heart health, the American Heart Association also provides important information, including the risk factors for heart disease, ways to reduce the factors you can control, warning signs for heart attack and stroke, and the science behind our recommendations.

With this newest edition of the *American Heart Association Healthy*

Fats, Low-Cholesterol Cookbook, we invite you to enjoy our classic favorite recipes, such as Tilapia Tacos with Roasted-Tomato Salsa (page 128) and Sirloin Steak with Portobello Mushrooms (page 189). We hope you'll also be inspired to try many of the new ones, such as Grilled Pizza with Grilled Vegetables (page 212) and Chicken Pot Pie with Mashed Potato Topping (page 172). As the perfect companion for today's healthy cook, this book will help you prepare wholesome meals so you and your family can eat wisely each and every day.

Rose Marie Robertson, M.D., FAHA, FACC
CHIEF SCIENCE AND MEDICAL OFFICER
American Heart Association/American Stroke Association

fats, cholesterol, and heart health

E ating well is one of the joys of life. Because you want foods that both taste good and are good for you, this cookbook offers many choices ranging from appetizers to desserts, all high in flavor but low in unhealthy nutrients including sodium, added sugars, saturated fat, and trans fat. Saturated and trans fats are dietary villains that cause blood levels of harmful low-density lipoprotein cholesterol (LDL, the "bad" cholesterol) to rise. That's a serious concern because higher levels of LDL cholesterol circulating in your blood are a major risk factor for heart disease.

You can take three important steps to help manage your risk of heart disease. First, evaluate your personal situation and identify all your risk factors. Second, take steps to control your LDL cholesterol level—and other risk factors—by making smart decisions about your diet and lifestyle. Third, commit to making good choices for the long term to live a longer, healthier life.

KNOW YOUR RISK

The first step is to assess your individual risk for heart disease. Risk factors are the behaviors and conditions that increase your chance of developing a disease. Some risk factors—aging, your medical history, and the medical history of your family—can't be changed. (For more information, see Appendix E on page 346.) Fortunately, many risk factors *can* be changed. Lifestyle choices such as smoking and physical inactivity, as well as conditions such as high blood cholesterol, high blood pressure, being overweight or obese, and diabetes, are all factors that you *can* do something about. In fact, heart disease is largely preventable. If you don't know your numbers for blood cholesterol, blood pressure, and blood glucose, visit your healthcare provider and find out what they are. Be sure to schedule regular visits with your healthcare provider to monitor your individual situation. Depending on your cholesterol levels and your other risk factors, decide together on target goals and the best approach for reaching them.

REDUCE YOUR RISK

By changing your habits, especially your dietary and lifestyle choices, you can help reduce your level of blood cholesterol as well as other risk factors. How much you have to modify your diet and lifestyle depends on several things, including your other risk factors and how your body responds to changes in your diet. For many people, relatively minor changes can reduce their risk significantly. Others need to make more extensive lifestyle changes. Eating well and being physically active are the best ways to control your LDL cholesterol level and other modifiable risk factors.

Eating a Heart-Healthy Diet

The more research we do, the more we understand how the foods we eat affect the levels of cholesterol in our blood. What actually is cholesterol? Cholesterol is a waxy substance that comes from two sources: your body and food. Your body, and especially your liver, makes all the cholesterol you need and circulates it through the blood. But cholesterol is also found in foods from animal sources, such as meat, poultry, and full-fat dairy products. Your liver produces more cholesterol when you eat a diet high in saturated and trans fats. That's why it's important to know what you're eating and what to cut back on to keep your blood cholesterol low. To achieve a heart-healthy diet, it's important to replace foods that are high in saturated fat and trans fat, as well as in sodium and added sugars, with nutritious foods.

Being Physically Active

In addition to eating nutritiously, we know that maintaining a healthy lifestyle—especially by staying physically active—is an important step to reduce your risk for heart disease and stroke. You can help lower your cholesterol primarily by getting regular exercise and managing your weight.

If your healthcare provider prescribes cholesterol-lowering drugs, you still should modify your diet and lifestyle. These changes not only lower cholesterol but also help control many of the other risk factors for heart disease, including high blood pressure, being overweight or obese, and diabetes.

COMMIT TO A LIFETIME OF HEALTHY CHOICES

Finally, managing your risk means committing to a lifestyle that promotes a longer, healthier life. If you eat wisely, stay physically active, take statins (if prescribed), and follow the recommendations of your healthcare provider, chances are you will:

- Reduce your likelihood of developing high blood cholesterol if you don't have it.
- Reduce your cholesterol levels if they are high.
- Reduce your risk of developing heart disease and having a stroke.

By consistently making healthy decisions throughout your life, you are taking an active role in managing your well-being. The smart choices you make today can bring long-lasting benefits to you and your family for many years to come.

healthy food, healthy heart

One of the best ways to take care of your heart is to understand the fundamentals of good nutrition and apply them in your everyday life. Once you have this information, you can build a heart-smart eating plan using our recipes and creatively adapting your own.

THE ESSENTIALS TO EATING WELL

As you plan your meals at home—and when you make food choices away from home—what matters most is to establish a well-balanced diet that provides variety among the food groups. If one day you eat too much of something you are trying to limit, be mindful of that and eat less in the following days to get back in balance. It is possible to satisfy your personal preferences and still be sure you get all the components of a healthy diet while limiting the less healthy foods.

Follow these basic nutrition guidelines for an overall healthy eating pattern:

- Eat lots of different fruits and vegetables.
- Make sure at least half of the grains you eat are whole-grain foods.
- Include fat-free and low-fat dairy products.
- Eat fish (especially those rich in omega-3 fatty acids) at least twice a week.

- Choose lean meats and poultry without skin and prepare them without added saturated and trans fats.
- Limit foods that contain "bad" fats (saturated and trans) and replace with those that contain "good" fats (mono-unsaturated and polyunsaturated).
- Choose and prepare foods with little or no salt.
- Reduce your consumption of beverages and foods with added sugars.

Fruits and Vegetables

Vegetables and fruits are great examples of nutrient-rich foods whether they are fresh, frozen, or canned. They are low in calories but provide important vitamins, minerals, fiber, and other nutrients. Try to eat the rainbow of fruits and vegetables to get the widest variety, such as (green) spinach, kale, collard greens, mustard greens, romaine lettuce; (red) tomatoes, beets, red bell pepper, raspberries; and (orange) carrots, sweet potatoes, pumpkins, mangoes, cantaloupes, apricots.

healthy hints

- Look for no-salt-added or low-sodium versions of canned vegetables and beans. Manufacturers continue to bring out new products to meet the demand for more-healthful choices.
- For canned fruits, read the ingredient labels to find options with the least amount of added sugar. Fruits that are canned in water are lower in calories than fruits canned in juice or syrup. Rinsing and draining both canned fruits and vegetables before you use them reduces sugar and sodium even further.

Grains

Any food made of wheat, rice, oats, corn, or another cereal is a grain product. Bread, pasta, oatmeal, and grits are all grain products. There are two main types of grain products: whole grains and refined grains. Try to eat whole-grain products for at least half of your daily servings.

Whole grains are high in fiber and complex carbohydrates and low in saturated fat, and they are a healthier choice than refined grains. Whole grains contain the entire grain—the bran, germ, and endosperm. Healthy choices include whole-wheat flour, oatmeal, corn, whole-grain cornmeal, brown rice, quinoa, buckwheat, wild rice, barley, bulgur, and whole-grain cereals and breads.

On the other hand, refined grains have been milled (ground into flour or meal), which results in the bran and germ being removed. This process removes much of the B vitamins, iron, and dietary fiber. Most refined grains are *enriched*, which means that some of the B vitamins and iron are added back after processing. Fiber, however, is not added back to enriched grains. Some sources of enriched grains are wheat flour, enriched bread, and white rice.

healthy hints

- To find grains in their whole form, look beyond the labeling on the packaging and read the ingredients list. When choosing a bread, cereal, or grain product, look for those that list the whole grain as the first ingredient on the label.
- Most commercial muffins, cakes, pies, doughnuts, and cookies are not made with whole grains, and they are high in calories and low in important nutrients. To enjoy these occasional treats, bake them at home using whole-wheat flour, unsaturated oils, and fruits or vegetables. For some

delicious ideas, see "Breads and Breakfast Dishes" (page 277) and "Desserts" (page 293).

- Commercial products are being reformulated to avoid the use of trans fat, but check nutrition labels for partially hydrogenated oils before you buy.

Dairy Products

Dairy foods are an important part of a healthy diet, providing calcium and protein. All adults ages 19 to 50 should aim to consume 1,000 milligrams of calcium each day (for maximal calcium retention). For adults ages 51 and older, that amount increases to 1,200 milligrams. Most healthcare providers encourage women in particular to eat fat-free and low-fat dairy products to get calcium. This helps reduce their risk of developing the bone disease osteoporosis. So many fat-free and low-fat dairy options are now available that you can easily avoid the high levels of saturated fat found in whole milk and whole-milk products. Healthy choices include fat-free or low-fat milk, cheeses, yogurt, sour cream, and cream cheese. To see the difference, take a look at the nutrition labels and compare a cup of whole milk to a cup of fat-free milk, for example. By choosing the fat-free version, you'll save about 65 calories and 4.5 grams of saturated fat.

healthy hints

- Keep in mind that many cheeses are high in saturated fat and that many fat-free or low-fat products have high levels of sodium and added sugars. Be sure to read the nutrition facts labels and compare products.

- If you're used to whole-milk products (3.5% fat), you may find it easier to taper off slowly. Try 1% low-fat milk first, then change to ½% low-fat milk. Soon you'll be able to switch to fat-free milk with no trouble.
- If you choose not to consume dairy products, other good sources of calcium include green vegetables such as spinach, kale, and broccoli, and some legumes and soybean products.

Fish and Seafood

Research suggests that increased intake of oily fish that contain omega-3 fatty acids—such as salmon, lake trout, herring, sardines, mackerel, and albacore tuna—reduces the risk of death from coronary artery disease. Aim to eat at least two servings of fish that's rich in omega-3 fatty acids every week. If you already have heart disease or high blood triglyceride levels, your healthcare professional may recommend fish oil supplements to help increase your intake of omega-3 fatty acids.

Shellfish, such as shrimp, squid, scallops, mussels, and clams, is low in saturated fat, so it's a good source of heart-healthy protein. There are also several tasty and healthy ways to prepare shellfish that don't add a lot of saturated and trans fats or sodium.

healthy hints

- Canned tuna is an easy way to get in omega-3s. Choose a very low sodium product and be sure it's packed in water or in a vacuum-sealed pouch.
- Although nearly all fish and shellfish may contain trace amounts of mercury or other contaminants, the health risks

from mercury exposure depend on the levels of mercury in the fish itself and the amount of seafood eaten. Eating a variety of fish will help minimize the possible adverse effects caused by pollutants in the environment. The FDA recommends that women who are pregnant, planning to become pregnant, or nursing—and young children—should avoid eating four types of fish with high mercury levels: tilefish from the Gulf of Mexico, shark, swordfish, and king mackerel. For most people, however, the benefits of eating fish far outweigh the risks.

- Choose low-sodium, low-fat seasonings, such as spices, herbs, and lemon juice, when you cook fish.

Poultry and Meat

Lean skinless poultry and lean meat are delicious sources of essential protein. Protein helps you to feel full and satisfied until your next meal, and it's critical for building muscle to keep you strong, especially as you grow older. The American Heart Association recommends consuming no more than 6 ounces of cooked lean skinless poultry or lean meat each day.

Healthy choices include skinless chicken and turkey, all cuts; lean beef cuts, such as sirloin, round steak, and rump roast; extra-lean ground beef; lean pork cuts, such as loin chops, tenderloin, and the lowest sodium available center-cut ham and Canadian bacon. Try to limit your consumption of red meat.

healthy hints

- Choose whole turkeys or turkey breasts that haven't been injected with broth or fats.
- Buy USDA Select grades of meat. They have less marbling than Prime or Choice.
- Be sure to discard any visible fat.
- When figuring serving sizes, remember that poultry (and meat) loses about 25 percent of its weight during cooking. (For example, 4 ounces of raw poultry [or meat] will weigh about 3 ounces when cooked.)
- Chill meat juices from cooking so you can easily skim off fat that hardens on the surface before you use those juices to make gravy, stews, or soups.
- Limit processed meats, such as bacon, hot dogs, bologna, salami, and sausage. They are often high in saturated fat and sodium. Reduced-fat, low-fat, and/or fat-free versions of these meats are available, but watch out for high sodium. Compare labels to find the brands that are lowest in calories, saturated fat, and sodium.
- Legumes, especially dried beans and peas, are also rich in fiber and provide protein. They are excellent alternatives to animal sources of protein that contain saturated fat. Also include a variety of legumes, such as green peas, black-eyed peas, chickpeas, kidney beans, navy beans, and lentils.

Fats and Oils

It's the type of fat more than how much fat you consume that most affects your blood cholesterol level. The main types of fat in foods are saturated fat, trans fat, and unsaturated fat. Saturated fats are found in animal products and in some tropical oils. Trans fat is found primarily in commercial products made with or fried in partially hydrogenated oils. Both of these types are the harmful fats and raise LDL cholesterol in the blood. Aim to get no more than 5 to 6 percent of calories from saturated fat and to reduce the percentage of calories from trans fat. For example, if you eat about 2,000 calories a day, you should limit your consumption of saturated fat to less than 13 grams (6 percent of 2,000 calories is 120 calories, divided by 9 calories, which are roughly equal to 1 gram of fat). You can find how much saturated fat is in foods by reading the nutritional analyses for recipes and reading the Nutrition Facts panels on food labels.

Focus on eating the better fats, polyunsaturated and monounsaturated, which are found in vegetable oils, nuts, and oily fish. Healthy choices include:

UNSATURATED OILS: canola, corn, olive, safflower, sesame, soybean, sunflower; salad dressings made with vegetable oils; light mayonnaise

LIQUID OR SOFT MARGARINES: The first ingredient on the food label should be unsaturated liquid vegetable oil rather than hydrogenated or partially hydrogenated oil; look for spreads made with vegetable oil.

NUTS AND SEEDS: Most nuts and any variety of seeds are high in helpful unsaturated fats. Check the food labels to compare varieties and select the product with the lowest sodium. Nuts and seeds are also high in calories, however, so adjust your intake according to your calorie needs.

OILY FISH: salmon, lake trout, herring, sardines, mackerel, and albacore tuna

One way to distinguish between the harmful ("bad") and helpful ("good") types of fats is to think in terms of their consistency. Fats and oils high in saturated fat tend to become hard at room temperature. On the other hand, oils that stay liquid at room temperature are high in polyunsaturated and monounsaturated fats. When it comes to fats, non-tropical liquid oils tend to have more of the better fats than do solid fats.

Changing oils from a liquid to a solid form, such as stick margarine, is done through the process of hydrogenation. This process creates harmful trans fat. Many food companies and restaurants have reformulated their products to reduce the amount of trans fats in foods or remove them completely. To reduce your intake of both saturated and trans fats, use liquid vegetable oil and trans-fat-free soft margarines instead of butter, stick margarine, or shortening.

healthy hints

- Choose products that are labeled "low in saturated fat," which means they contain no more than 1 gram of saturated fat per serving.
- Liquid and soft margarines in tubs work well for cooking and for flavoring vegetables and casseroles. Because they contain water, they are not recommended for most baking, however.
- Use cooking sprays—plain or flavored—in place of butter or oil on equipment such as pans, baking sheets, and casserole dishes. (Certain nonstick cookware manufacturers advise against using commercial sprays, which contain propellant. Be sure to check your warranty information.)
- Check nutrition labels for trans fat values, but be equally careful about saturated fat. Foods labeled "trans-fat-free" may still contain high amounts of saturated fat.

Sodium

Despite the widespread impression that most of the sodium we consume comes from the salt shaker, the reality is that more than 75 percent of the sodium in the average American diet comes from salt added to packaged and processed foods. Eating too much sodium is linked to high blood pressure, a condition commonly found in people with high cholesterol. Eating a healthy diet, being physically active, and limiting your sodium intake are important steps to managing your blood pressure. To lower your blood pressure, eat no more than 2,400 mg of sodium per day. Reducing your daily sodium intake to 1,500 mg is desirable because it is associated with even greater reductions in blood pressure.

healthy hints

- Read food labels and always look for products with the lowest sodium available.
- Cook more at home and use salt-free seasoning blends and no-sodium flavor enhancers, such as fresh citrus juices, herbs, garlic, and chiles.
- If you dine out, check out the restaurant menu before you go to help you make wiser choices and avoid dishes made with sodium-heavy ingredients, such as deli or processed meats, cheeses, sauces, condiments, and bread.

Added Sugars

Sugars in your diet can be naturally occurring or added. Naturally occurring sugars are found *naturally* in foods such as fruit (fructose) and milk (lactose). Added sugars are sugars and syrups put in foods during preparation or processing, or added at the table. The major sources of added sugars are regular soft drinks, pastries, candy, desserts, and fruit drinks (fruitades and fruit punch). Many people consume more sugar than they realize. It's important to be aware of how much sugar you consume because our bodies don't need sugar to function properly. Added sugars contribute zero nutrients but many added calories that can lead to extra pounds or even obesity, thereby reducing heart health.

The American Heart Association recommends limiting the amount of added sugars you consume to no more than half of your daily discretionary calories allowance. For most American women, that's no more than 100 calories per day, or about 6 teaspoons (24 grams) of sugar. For men, it's 150 calories per day, or about 9 teaspoons (36 grams).

healthy hints

- Cut back on the amount of sugar added to things you eat or drink regularly like cereal, pancakes, coffee, or tea. Try cutting the usual amount of sugar you add by half and wean down from there.
- Swap out the soda for sugar-free or low-calorie beverages. However, water is always the best choice. Infuse it with fresh citrus to make it more appealing.
- Eat fresh, frozen, dried, or canned fruits in place of sugary desserts. Choose fruit canned in water or natural juice. Avoid fruit canned in syrup, especially heavy syrup. Rinse and drain canned fruit in a colander to remove excess syrup or juice.
- Reduce the sugar in recipes. When baking cookies, brownies, or cakes, cut the sugar called for in your recipe by one-third to one-half. Often you won't notice the difference.
- Instead of adding sugar in recipes, use flavorful extracts like almond, vanilla, orange, or lemon.

- Enhance foods with spices instead of sugar. Try ginger, allspice, cinnamon, or nutmeg, all of which are considered sweet spices.

PORTION CONTROL

As part of an overall healthy eating plan, it's important to know not only what to eat but also how much to eat. Recognizing reasonable serving sizes and applying that information is critical in maintaining a weight that's healthy for you. It's not as hard as it may seem. Try to visualize healthy servings of the foods you typically eat the most. To do this, think in terms of the size of common objects:

- 3 ounces of cooked meat, poultry, or fish is the size of a computer mouse.
- 3 ounces of cooked fish is about the size of a checkbook.
- 1 teaspoon of soft margarine is the size of 1 die.
- 1½ ounces of cheese is the size of a 1½-inch cube.
- 1 medium baked potato is the size of an average fist.
- 1-cup servings or a medium piece of fruit is the size of a baseball.
- ½ cup servings are the size of half a baseball.
- Half of a bagel is about the size of a hockey puck.

Use the chart on the following page as a guide to help you choose foods and plan the amounts to serve.

FOOD TYPE	EXAMPLES OF HEALTHY SERVING SIZES
Breads, Cereals, and Grains Whole-grain breads and cereals, pasta (especially whole grain), rice (brown and white), potatoes, and fat-free, low-sodium whole-grain crackers	1 slice bread 1 cup cereal flakes ½ cup cooked rice, pasta, or potato 5 crackers
Vegetables and Legumes (Dried Beans, Peas, and Lentils) Fresh, frozen, canned—without added saturated fat, sauce, or salt	1 cup leafy or raw vegetable ½ cup cooked vegetable or legume
Fruits Fresh, frozen, canned, or dried—without added sugar	1 medium piece fruit ½ cup diced fruit ¾ cup fruit juice
Dairy Products Fat-free or low-fat milk, buttermilk, yogurt, sour cream, cream cheese, and cheese (with no more than 3 grams of saturated fat per ounce, such as low-fat cottage cheese)	1 cup milk 1 cup yogurt 1½ ounces cheese ½ cup cottage cheese
Fats and Oils Unsaturated, nontropical vegetable oils, liquid or soft margarines and vegetable oil spreads, salad dressings, nuts, and seeds	1 teaspoon soft margarine or vegetable oil 1 tablespoon regular salad dressing or 2 tablespoons low-fat dressing 1 ounce nuts or seeds
Meat, Poultry, and Seafood Lean cuts of loin, leg, round; lean ground meat; skinless poultry; fish	3 ounces or less of cooked meat, poultry, and seafood

healthy lifestyle,
healthy heart

The message is simple: Regular physical activity protects against heart disease; it helps to reduce your cholesterol and blood pressure levels and manage your weight. In addition to the health benefits you'll gain from being active, you'll probably find you feel better, have more energy, and can make other lifestyle changes more easily.

STAY ACTIVE

For overall cardiovascular health, the American Heart Association suggests at least 150 minutes of moderately intense physical activity per week or 75 minutes of vigorous physical activity per week and muscle strengthening activity at least twice per week. Thirty minutes a day, five times a week is an easy goal to remember. If you're trying to lower your blood pressure and cholesterol, the American Heart Association recommends an average of 40 minutes of moderate- to vigorous-intensity aerobic activity three to four times per week. You can break your activity into sessions of 10 minutes or more and include moderate-intensity activities you might not consider "exercise," such as gardening and housework, which add up during the day.

Use the table on the following page to estimate how many calories you can burn in various activities at different intensities. Keep in mind that your gender and current weight affect the number of calories you use, and that the more muscular you are, the more calories you burn. The numbers given are for a person of about 150 pounds. If you weigh more, you will burn more, and if you weigh less, you will burn fewer calories.

PHYSICAL ACTIVITY	CALORIES BURNED IN 30 MINUTES
Moderate Intensity	
Hiking	185
Light gardening/yard work	165
Dancing	165
Golf (walking and carrying clubs)	165
Bicycling (less than 10 mph)	145
Walking (3.5 mph)	140
Weight lifting (light workout)	110
Stretching	90
Vigorous Intensity	
Running/jogging	295
Bicycling (more than 10 mph)	295
Swimming (slow freestyle laps)	255
Aerobics	240
Walking (4.5 mph)	230
Weight lifting (vigorous workout)	220
Basketball (vigorous)	220

It's a good idea to talk with your healthcare provider before starting an exercise program if you haven't exercised for a long time. Likewise, if you have had a heart attack or have a medical condition (such as high blood pressure, high cholesterol, diabetes, or obesity), take prescription medication, are a smoker, are over 65, or are at risk for heart disease because of family history, it's important to discuss your individual situation with your healthcare professional.

MANAGE YOUR WEIGHT

It's one thing to read about what you "should" do to stay healthy, but it's another to decide to make those recommendations a real part of your life. Recognizing the habits that keep you from effectively managing your weight will help you adopt healthier behaviors that lead to a longer, stronger life.

Each of us needs an ideal number of calories to maintain a healthy weight. You can estimate how many daily calories you need based on your age, gender, and level of physical activity. Remember that as you age, you'll need fewer calories to maintain your weight even if you stay at the same level of activity.

ACTIVITY LEVEL AND ESTIMATED CALORIES BURNED			
Age, Years	Sedentary	Moderately Active	Active
Female			
19–30	1,800–2,000	2,000–2,200	2,400
31–50	1,800	2,000	2,200
51+	1,600	1,800	2,000–2,200
Male			
19–30	2,400–2,600	2,600–2,800	3,000
31–50	2,200–2,400	2,400–2,600	2,800–3,000
51+	2,000–2,200	2,200–2,400	2,400–2,800

SEDENTARY means you have a lifestyle that includes only the light physical activity associated with typical day-to-day life.

MODERATELY ACTIVE means you have a lifestyle that includes physical activity equivalent to walking about 1.5 to 3 miles per day at 3 to 4 miles per hour, in addition to the light physical activity associated with typical day-to-day life.

ACTIVE means you have a lifestyle that includes physical activity equivalent to walking more than 3 miles per day at 3 to 4 miles per hour, in addition to the light physical activity associated with typical day-to-day life.

Maintain the Calorie Balance That's Right for You

To avoid weight gain, you should burn at least as many calories as you eat every day. Calories *in* should equal calories *out*. If you consistently take in more calories than you need for your age and level of physical activity, you will gradually gain weight. The table on the previous page should give you an idea of what you need to maintain your calorie balance.

Know When to Lose Weight

Being overweight or obese increases your likelihood of developing heart disease and stroke even if you have no other risk factors. Excess weight reduces levels of helpful HDL cholesterol and may raise levels of harmful LDL cholesterol. The way weight is distributed on your body may be a clue to your risk of heart disease. Your risk is significantly greater if you're a man with a waist measuring more than 40 inches or a woman with a waist more than 35 inches. Losing weight—even as little as 3 to 5 percent of your body weight—can help reduce your LDL cholesterol levels.

You can use the body mass index (BMI) as a starting place to see whether you are considered underweight, normal weight, overweight, or obese. This standard method classifies body weight based on your weight and height. If the table on the following page indicates that you fall in the obese category or that you fall in the overweight category and have other risk factors, discuss your BMI number with your healthcare provider, who will determine what a healthy weight is for you. Avoid gaining weight if you are a normal weight or you are overweight without additional risk factors. To best manage your weight, eat the right amount of calories for you and participate in regular physical activity.

To find your BMI:

- Weigh yourself without clothes or shoes. Measure your height without shoes.
- Find your height in the left-hand column of the chart on the following page and find the range into which your weight falls.

BODY MASS INDEX			
Height	Minimal Risk (BMI under 25)	Overweight (BMI 25.0-29.9)	Obese (BMI 30.0+)
4'10"	118 lb or less	119-142 lb	143 lb or more
4'11"	123	124-147	148
5'0"	127	128-152	153
5'1"	131	132-157	158
5'2"	135	136-163	164
5'3"	140	141-168	169
5'4"	144	145-173	174
5'5"	149	150-179	180
5'6"	154	155-185	186
5'7"	158	159-190	191
5'8"	163	164-196	197
5'9"	168	169-202	203
5'10"	173	174-208	209
5'11"	178	179-214	215
6'0"	183	184-220	221
6'1"	188	189-226	227
6'2"	193	194-232	233
6'3"	199	200-239	240
6'4"	204	205-245	246

BELOW 25—A BMI from 18.5 to 24.9 is considered healthy. BMI values less than 18.5 are considered underweight.

25.0 TO 29.9—Overweight—A BMI in this range indicates a moderate risk of heart and blood vessel disease. A BMI of 25 translates to about 10 percent over ideal body weight.

30 OR MORE—Obese—A BMI over 30 indicates a high risk of heart and blood vessel disease.

DON'T SMOKE, AND AVOID SECONDHAND SMOKE

If you smoke, ask your doctor about the best ways to quit. When you stop smoking, your risk for heart disease and stroke drops rapidly.

DRINK ALCOHOL IN MODERATION—IF AT ALL

Studies have shown that a moderate intake of alcohol may reduce risk for heart disease. Drinking in moderation means no more than one drink per day for women or two drinks per day for men. One drink is equal to 12 ounces of beer, 5 ounces of wine, or 1½ ounces of 80-proof distilled spirits.

At the same time, the many dangerous effects of high alcohol intake—such as high blood pressure, heart failure, and an increased caloric intake—can far outweigh the benefits. Alcohol also adds calories to your diet without adding nutrients. If you do drink alcohol, do so in moderation. If you don't drink, don't start.

SCHEDULE REGULAR DOCTOR VISITS

The American Heart Association recommends all adults age 20 or older who have not been diagnosed with cardiovascular disease to have their cholesterol checked every four to six years as part of an overall risk assessment. However, be sure to check with your healthcare professional about what's best for *you*.

recipes

Each recipe in the book includes a nutritional analysis so you can decide how that dish fits with your dietary needs. These guidelines will give you some details on how the analyses were calculated.

- Each analysis is for a *single* serving; garnishes or optional ingredients are *not* included unless noted.
- Because of the many variables involved, the nutrient values provided should be considered approximate. When figuring portions, remember that the serving sizes are approximate also.
- When ingredient options are listed, the first one is analyzed. When a range of amount is given, the average is analyzed.
- Values other than fats are rounded to the nearest whole number. Fat values are rounded to the nearest half gram. Because of the rounding, values for saturated, trans, mono-unsaturated, and polyunsaturated fats may not add up to the amount shown for total fat value.
- All the recipes are analyzed using unsalted or low-sodium ingredients whenever possible. In some cases, we call for unprocessed foods or no-salt-added and low-sodium products, then add table salt sparingly for flavor. If only a regular commercial product is available, we use the one with the lowest sodium.
- We specify canola, corn, and olive oils in these recipes, but you can also use other heart-healthy unsaturated oils, such as safflower, soybean, and sunflower.

- Meats are analyzed as lean, with all visible fat discarded. Values for ground beef are based on lean meat that is 95 percent fat free.
- When meat, poultry, or seafood is marinated and the marinade is discarded, the analysis includes all of the sodium from the marinade but none of the other nutrients from it.
- If alcohol is used in a cooked dish, we estimate that most of the alcohol calories evaporate as the food cooks.
- Because product labeling in the marketplace can vary and change quickly, we use the generic terms "fat-free" and "low-fat" throughout to avoid confusion.
- We use the abbreviations *g* for gram and *mg* for milligram.

Appetizers, Snacks, and Beverages

CREAMY CAPER DIP 30

ROASTED RED BELL PEPPER DIP 31

SMOKED SALMON DIP WITH CUCUMBER AND HERBS 32

SWEET-SPICE VANILLA DIP WITH DRIED PLUMS AND PECANS 33

FRESH BASIL AND KALAMATA HUMMUS 34

SOUTHWESTERN BLACK BEAN SPREAD 35

ZUCCHINI SPREAD 36

TOMATO BURSTS 37

TRAIL MIX WITH COCOA-DUSTED ALMONDS 38

NECTARINE-PLUM CHUTNEY 39

ORANGE-GINGER CHICKEN SKEWERS 40

CANAPÉS WITH ROASTED GARLIC, ARTICHOKE, AND CHÈVRE SPREAD 41

ZESTY POTATO SKINS 42

KALE-AND-HAM-STUFFED CREMINI MUSHROOMS 44

BANANA MINI SNACK CAKES 45

SANGRÍA-STYLE POMEGRANATE COOLERS 46

ORANGE-STRAWBERRY FROTH 47

PINEAPPLE SHAKE 48

SPICED APPLE CIDER 49

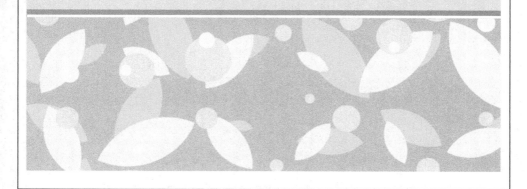

Creamy Caper Dip

Serves 12

Elegant yet so easy, this peppy dip can be used as a rich topping to perk up the simplicity of cucumber or tomato slices; or serve it as a sauce with grilled salmon.

- 8 ounces fat-free plain yogurt
- ¼ cup light mayonnaise
- 2½ tablespoons capers, drained
- 2 tablespoons Dijon mustard (lowest sodium available)
- 1 medium garlic clove, minced
- 1 tablespoon olive oil (extra virgin preferred)

In a food processor or blender, process all the ingredients except the oil until smooth. Transfer to a small serving bowl.

Stir in the oil. Cover and refrigerate until serving time, up to 8 hours. Stir before serving.

PER SERVING

Calories 36	Cholesterol 2 mg	DIETARY EXCHANGES:
Total Fat 2.5 g	Sodium 162 mg	½ fat
Saturated Fat 0.5 g	Carbohydrates 2 g	
Trans Fat 0.0 g	Fiber 0 g	
Polyunsaturated Fat 1.0 g	Sugars 2 g	
Monounsaturated Fat 1.0 g	Protein 1 g	

Roasted Red Bell Pepper Dip

Serves 16

A little kick from cayenne and a hint of smokiness from paprika bring the party to life with this appetizer. Add a creative flair to any celebration by serving it in hollowed-out red, green, and/or yellow bell peppers.

- 1 cup fat-free sour cream
- 1 7-ounce jar roasted red bell peppers in water, drained
- ¼ cup coarsely chopped fresh dillweed
- ¼ teaspoon garlic powder
- ¼ teaspoon cayenne or crushed red pepper flakes
- ¼ teaspoon smoked paprika
- ⅛ teaspoon salt
- 3 tablespoons dried minced onion

In a food processor or blender, process all the ingredients except the onion for 30 seconds, or until smooth. Transfer to a small serving bowl.

Stir in the onion. Cover and refrigerate for 30 minutes, or until serving time. Stir before serving.

....

COOK'S TIP ON SMOKED PAPRIKA: Smoked over wood planks, then ground into powder, sweet red bell peppers become smoked paprika and add both color and flavor to foods from soup to nuts.

....

PER SERVING

Calories 20	Cholesterol 3 mg	DIETARY EXCHANGES:
Total Fat 0.0 g	Sodium 54 mg	Free
Saturated Fat 0.0 g	Carbohydrates 4 g	
Trans Fat 0.0 g	Fiber 0 g	
Polyunsaturated Fat 0.0 g	Sugars 1 g	
Monounsaturated Fat 0.0 g	Protein 1 g	

Smoked Salmon Dip with Cucumber and Herbs

Serves 16

Creamy and cool but with a slight smoky flavor, this dip is hard to resist. Surround a bowl of it with bell pepper strips, baby carrots, celery sticks, and halved cherry tomatoes for an eye-catching presentation.

1 medium cucumber, peeled and diced
1 cup fat-free sour cream
2 ounces smoked salmon (not lox; lowest sodium available), rinsed with cold water, patted dry, and diced
1 tablespoon chopped fresh dillweed or 1 teaspoon dried dillweed, crumbled
1 teaspoon grated lemon zest
1 tablespoon fresh lemon juice
1 teaspoon finely chopped green onions (green part only)
¼ teaspoon paprika

In a small serving bowl, stir together all the ingredients except the paprika. Smooth the surface of the dip.

Sprinkle with the paprika. Serve immediately or cover and refrigerate for up to two days to serve chilled.

....

COOK'S TIP ON SMOKED SALMON: When shopping for smoked salmon, read the nutrition labels and choose the product with the lowest sodium. Rinsing the salmon under cold water before use helps remove some of the excess sodium.

....

PER SERVING

Calories 19	Cholesterol 3 mg	DIETARY EXCHANGES:
Total Fat 0.0 g	Sodium 82 mg	Free
Saturated Fat 0.0 g	Carbohydrates 3 g	
Trans Fat 0.0 g	Fiber 0 g	
Polyunsaturated Fat 0.0 g	Sugars 1 g	
Monounsaturated Fat 0.0 g	Protein 2 g	

Sweet-Spice Vanilla Dip with Dried Plums and Pecans

Serves 8

Creamy vanilla yogurt, sweet spices, dried plums, and toasted pecans create a heavenly combo. Try apple slices, strawberries, pineapple chunks, or low-fat gingersnaps as dippers.

> 2 **tablespoons chopped pecans**
> **Cooking spray**
> 1 **teaspoon light brown sugar**
> ⅛ **teaspoon ground nutmeg**
> 6 **ounces fat-free vanilla yogurt**
> ½ **teaspoon ground cinnamon**
> ⅛ **teaspoon ground ginger**
> 3 **ounces dried plums, chopped**

Put the pecans in a small skillet. Lightly spray with cooking spray. Sprinkle the brown sugar and nutmeg over the pecans. Cook over medium heat for 1 to 2 minutes, or until the brown sugar is dissolved and slightly caramelized on the pecans, stirring constantly. Transfer to a small plate and let cool for about 5 minutes.

Meanwhile, in a small serving bowl, whisk together the yogurt, cinnamon, and ginger. Stir in the plums.

If serving immediately, sprinkle the dip with the pecans. If serving chilled, cover and refrigerate the dip for up to four days without the pecans. Store the pecans in an airtight container at room temperature. Just before serving, sprinkle the dip with the pecans.

....

COOK'S TIP: To cut dried plums or other sticky foods easily, use kitchen scissors lightly sprayed with cooking spray.

....

PER SERVING

Calories 58	Cholesterol 0 mg	DIETARY EXCHANGES:
Total Fat 1.5 g	Sodium 16 mg	½ other carbohydrate
Saturated Fat 0.0 g	Carbohydrates 11 g	
Trans Fat 0.0 g	Fiber 1 g	
Polyunsaturated Fat 0.5 g	Sugars 8 g	
Monounsaturated Fat 0.5 g	Protein 2 g	

Fresh Basil and Kalamata Hummus

Serves 14

What better partners for the creaminess of pureed white beans than the lush taste of fresh basil and the lingering briny taste of kalamata olives?

1	15.5-ounce can no-salt-added cannellini beans, rinsed and drained
½	cup tightly packed fresh basil, coarsely chopped
½	cup fat-free sour cream
12	pitted kalamata olives
2	tablespoons olive oil (extra virgin preferred)
1	medium garlic clove, minced
¼	teaspoon salt

In a food processor or blender, process all the ingredients until smooth. Transfer to a small serving bowl.

PER SERVING

		DIETARY EXCHANGES:
Calories 60	Cholesterol 1 mg	½ starch
Total Fat 3.0 g	Sodium 111 mg	½ fat
Saturated Fat 0.5 g	Carbohydrates 6 g	
Trans Fat 0.0 g	Fiber 1 g	
Polyunsaturated Fat 0.5 g	Sugars 1 g	
Monounsaturated Fat 2.0 g	Protein 2 g	

Southwestern Black Bean Spread

Serves 12

Serve this zesty mixture on crisp jícama sticks, toasted whole-grain pita bread, or unsalted baked tortilla chips. For a speedy snack on the run, use it as a topping for a warm corn tortilla. You can just roll it up and go.

- 1 **15.5-ounce can no-salt-added black beans, rinsed and drained**
- 1 **4-ounce can diced green chiles, drained**
- ½ **cup roasted red bell peppers, drained if bottled**
- 2 **tablespoons fresh lime juice and 1 tablespoon fresh lime juice, divided use**
- 2 **medium garlic cloves, minced**
- 1 **teaspoon ground cumin**
- 1 **teaspoon onion powder**
- ¼ **teaspoon salt**
- ½ **cup fat-free sour cream**
- 1 **large tomato, diced**
- 1 **small avocado, diced**

In a food processor or blender, process the beans, chiles, roasted peppers, 2 tablespoons lime juice, the garlic, cumin, onion powder, and salt until the desired texture. Spread on a serving plate or in a shallow bowl.

In a small bowl, whisk together the sour cream and the remaining 1 tablespoon lime juice. Dollop the mixture onto the bean spread or lightly smooth it over the bean spread.

Sprinkle with the tomato and avocado.

....

COOK'S TIP ON AVOCADOS: Look for avocados that are heavy for their size and yield to gentle pressure. If you have an avocado that feels too firm, let it ripen on the counter for a couple of days, or put it in a brown paper bag with a tomato or an apple to speed up the process.

....

PER SERVING

Calories 60	Cholesterol 2 mg	DIETARY EXCHANGES:
Total Fat 1.0 g	Sodium 98 mg	½ starch
Saturated Fat 0.0 g	Carbohydrates 10 g	
Trans Fat 0.0 g	Fiber 2 g	
Polyunsaturated Fat 0.0 g	Sugars 2 g	
Monounsaturated Fat 0.5 g	Protein 3 g	

Zucchini Spread

Serves 8

Serve this versatile, nut-studded spread with salt-free, whole-wheat crackers or vegetable sticks. For a change-of-pace sandwich, lightly coat the inside of a whole-grain pita pocket with the spread, then stuff the pita with your favorite vegetables.

3½ cups shredded unpeeled zucchini, squeezed in paper towels to remove the excess liquid
¼ cup finely chopped fresh parsley or cilantro
2 tablespoons red wine vinegar
1 tablespoon olive oil (extra virgin preferred)
1 medium garlic clove, minced
¼ teaspoon salt
Pepper to taste
2 tablespoons finely chopped walnuts or pecans, dry-roasted

In a food processor or blender, process all the ingredients except the walnuts until smooth. Transfer to a small serving bowl.

Fold in the walnuts. Cover and refrigerate until serving time.

COOK'S TIP ON DRY-ROASTING NUTS AND SEEDS ON THE STOVETOP: Don't be tempted to skip the dry-roasting step here and in many other recipes. Even though only a small amount of nuts is used, the roasting brings out tremendous flavor. Spread the nuts in a single layer in a skillet. Dry-roast over medium heat for about 4 minutes, or just until fragrant, stirring frequently. Watch carefully so they don't burn.

PER SERVING

Calories 36	Cholesterol 0 mg	DIETARY EXCHANGES:
Total Fat 3.0 g	Sodium 76 mg	½ fat
Saturated Fat 0.5 g	Carbohydrates 2 g	
Trans Fat 0.0 g	Fiber 1 g	
Polyunsaturated Fat 1.0 g	Sugars 1 g	
Monounsaturated Fat 1.5 g	Protein 1 g	

Tomato Bursts

Serves 8

Hollowed-out cherry tomatoes taste extra good when they're filled with Mediterranean-inspired creaminess.

- 2 **ounces low-fat cream cheese**
- 12 **kalamata olives, finely chopped**
- 3 **tablespoons minced green onions**
- 1 **teaspoon dried basil, crumbled**
- 1 **medium garlic clove, minced**
- ⅛ **teaspoon salt**
- 32 **cherry tomatoes**

In a small bowl, stir together all the ingredients except the tomatoes.

Cut a thin slice from the top of each tomato. Using a ¼-teaspoon measuring spoon, scoop out and discard the pulp. (To remove any remaining seeds or loose pulp, run the tomatoes under cold water and drain upside down on paper towels.) Fill each tomato with about 1 teaspoon of the cream cheese mixture. Transfer to a platter. Cover and refrigerate until serving time, up to 8 hours.

PER SERVING

Calories 48	Cholesterol 5 mg	DIETARY EXCHANGES:
Total Fat 3.5 g	Sodium 158 mg	1 vegetable
Saturated Fat 1.0 g	Carbohydrates 4 g	½ fat
Trans Fat 0.0 g	Fiber 1 g	
Polyunsaturated Fat 0.5 g	Sugars 2 g	
Monounsaturated Fat 1.5 g	Protein 1 g	

Trail Mix with Cocoa-Dusted Almonds

Serves 12

Need an energy boost before your workout? Just grab a handful of this sweet-and-crunchy fuel on your way to the gym or soccer practice.

2 tablespoons unsweetened cocoa powder
2 teaspoons brown sugar
½ cup whole almonds
1 teaspoon honey
½ teaspoon vanilla extract
½ cup dried apricots, quartered
½ cup dates, halved
½ cup unsalted walnut halves, dry-roasted
½ cup unsalted peanuts, dry-roasted
¼ cup unsalted sunflower seeds, dry-roasted
¼ cup raisins

In a small bowl, stir together the cocoa powder and brown sugar. In a small skillet, heat the almonds, honey, and vanilla over very low heat for 1 to 2 minutes, or until the honey has melted and the almonds are sticky, stirring constantly. Add the almonds to the cocoa powder mixture, stirring to coat well. Pour the almonds into a fine-mesh sieve, shaking gently to remove the excess coating.

In a large bowl, stir together the almonds and the remaining ingredients. Transfer to a tightly covered container. Store in a cool, dry place at room temperature for up to one week.

....

COOK'S TIP ON DRY-ROASTING NUTS AND SEEDS IN THE OVEN: To dry-roast a large amount of nuts or seeds at one time, place them in a shallow baking dish. Roast them at 350°F for 10 to 15 minutes, stirring occasionally. You can freeze them in an airtight container or resealable plastic freezer bag so they can be ready at a moment's notice. You don't even need to thaw them.

....

PER SERVING

Calories 166	Cholesterol 0 mg	DIETARY EXCHANGES:
Total Fat 11.0 g	Sodium 3 mg	1 fruit
Saturated Fat 1.0 g	Carbohydrates 17 g	1 lean meat
Trans Fat 0.0 g	Fiber 3 g	1½ fat
Polyunsaturated Fat 4.5 g	Sugars 12 g	
Monounsaturated Fat 4.0 g	Protein 5 g	

Nectarine-Plum Chutney

Serves 6

To serve this sweet-and-sour chutney as an appetizer, use it to top salt-free crackers lightly spread with low-fat cream cheese. A lively condiment that's especially tasty with curried dishes, such as Creamy Chicken Curry (page 158) or Quick Curry-Baked Chicken with Cucumber Raita (page 148), this chutney also pairs beautifully with almost any grilled or roasted entrée.

> 3 small plums, diced
> 1 medium Granny Smith apple, peeled and diced
> 1 medium nectarine, diced
> ¼ cup sugar
> ¼ small onion, diced
> ¼ medium red bell pepper, diced
> ¼ cup cider vinegar
> 2 tablespoons golden raisins
> 1 teaspoon grated orange zest
> ⅛ teaspoon salt
> ⅛ teaspoon ground nutmeg

In a medium stainless steel, enameled steel, or nonstick saucepan, stir together all the ingredients. Cook over medium-high heat for 3 to 4 minutes, or until the sugar dissolves, stirring occasionally. Reduce the heat and simmer for 40 to 45 minutes, or until the fruit is tender, stirring occasionally. Let cool. Transfer to a serving bowl. Cover and refrigerate until serving time.

PER SERVING

Calories 87	Cholesterol 0 mg	DIETARY EXCHANGES:
Total Fat 0.5 g	Sodium 50 mg	1 fruit
Saturated Fat 0.0 g	Carbohydrates 22 g	½ other carbohydrate
Trans Fat 0.0 g	Fiber 2 g	
Polyunsaturated Fat 0.0 g	Sugars 19 g	
Monounsaturated Fat 0.0 g	Protein 1 g	

Orange-Ginger Chicken Skewers

Serves 10

This triple-hitter barbecue sauce does triple the work as it's used in the basting, finishing, and dipping sauces for these broiled chicken strips. It infuses the juicy chicken with the flavors of berries, citrus, and ginger.

Cooking spray

12 ounces boneless, skinless chicken breasts, all visible fat discarded, cut into 40 thin strips

½ cup barbecue sauce (lowest sodium available)

¼ cup all-fruit blackberry spread

2 teaspoons grated orange zest

1 teaspoon grated peeled gingerroot

Soak twenty 6- to 8-inch wooden skewers in cold water for at least 10 minutes to keep them from charring, or use metal skewers.

Preheat the broiler. Lightly spray the broiler pan and rack with cooking spray.

Thread 2 chicken strips onto each skewer in an "s" shape.

In a small bowl, whisk together the remaining ingredients until smooth. If the spread is too lumpy, microwave on 100 percent power (high) for 30 seconds, or until smooth, stirring once halfway through. Divide the sauce as follows: half in a small bowl for the basting sauce, one-fourth in the original bowl for the finishing sauce, and the remaining one-fourth in a small serving bowl for the dipping sauce.

Baste the chicken with about half the basting sauce.

Broil the chicken about 4 inches from the heat for 2 minutes. Turn over the chicken. Using a clean basting brush, baste with the remaining basting sauce. Broil for 2 minutes, or until the chicken is no longer pink in the center. Using a clean basting brush, baste the chicken with the finishing sauce.

Transfer the skewers to a platter. Serve with the reserved dipping sauce.

PER SERVING

Calories 79	Cholesterol 22 mg	DIETARY EXCHANGES:
Total Fat 1.0 g	Sodium 124 mg	½ other carbohydrate
Saturated Fat 0.0 g	Carbohydrates 9 g	1 lean meat
Trans Fat 0.0 g	Fiber 0 g	
Polyunsaturated Fat 0.0 g	Sugars 8 g	
Monounsaturated Fat 0.5 g	Protein 7 g	

40 HEALTHY FATS, LOW-CHOLESTEROL COOKBOOK

Canapés with Roasted Garlic, Artichoke, and Chèvre Spread

Serves 18

You might want to make a double batch of these simple but sophisticated appetizers, which are sure to be a favorite at your next gathering. Crisp toasted pita wedges are the perfect base for a creamy goat cheese mixture, which is then topped with juicy cherry tomato halves.

> 6 medium garlic cloves, unpeeled
> 6 7-inch whole-grain pita breads, each cut into sixths
> 9 ounces frozen artichoke hearts, thawed and chopped
> ½ cup light mayonnaise
> 2 ounces soft goat cheese
> ⅛ teaspoon pepper (white preferred)
> 2 tablespoons thinly sliced green onions (green part only)
> 18 cherry tomatoes, halved lengthwise

Preheat the oven to 350°F.

Put the garlic in a garlic roaster or small ovenproof pan and place on the bottom oven rack. Bake for 5 minutes.

Arrange the pitas in a single layer on a baking sheet.

After the garlic has baked for 5 minutes, place the baking sheet with the pitas on the middle oven rack. Bake for 10 minutes. Transfer the garlic and pitas to cooling racks and let cool for 10 minutes, leaving the oven on.

Discard the stem ends of the garlic. Squeeze the baked garlic onto a cutting board, discarding the peel. Mince the garlic. Transfer to a medium bowl.

Stir in the artichokes, mayonnaise, goat cheese, and pepper.

Spread about 1 teaspoon garlic mixture over each pita wedge. Sprinkle with the green onions. Press a cherry tomato half with the cut side up into the garlic mixture. Arrange in a single layer on the baking sheet. Bake for 5 minutes. Serve immediately.

PER SERVING

Calories 96	Cholesterol 4 mg	DIETARY EXCHANGES:
Total Fat 3.0 g	Sodium 200 mg	1 starch
Saturated Fat 0.5 g	Carbohydrates 15 g	½ fat
Trans Fat 0.0 g	Fiber 3 g	
Polyunsaturated Fat 1.5 g	Sugars 1 g	
Monounsaturated Fat 0.5 g	Protein 3 g	

Zesty Potato Skins

Serves 8

These filled potato skins are perfect football-watching snacks. Spiced with southwestern flair, they're an appealing alternative to the all-too-familiar chips and dip.

      6 **medium red potatoes (about 1¼ pounds total)**
         Cooking spray
      ½ **teaspoon garlic powder**
      ½ **teaspoon chili powder and ¼ teaspoon chili powder, divided use**
      ½ **teaspoon ground cumin**
      ⅛ **teaspoon pepper**
      8 **ounces fat-free cottage cheese, undrained**
      ½ **teaspoon grated lime zest**
   1½ **tablespoons fresh lime juice**
      1 **tablespoon finely chopped green onions (green part only)**
      4 **large black olives, each cut into 6 slices**

Preheat the oven to 450°F.

Wrap each potato in aluminum foil. Transfer to a baking sheet. Bake for 1 hour, or until the potatoes are tender when pierced with the tip of a sharp knife. Remove from the oven.

Unwrap the potatoes and let stand until cool enough to handle. Cut each potato in half. Scoop out the pulp, leaving a ¼-inch border of the shell all the way around. Halve each half. Lightly spray the pulp side with cooking spray.

In a small bowl, stir together the garlic powder, ½ teaspoon chili powder, the cumin, and pepper. Sprinkle on the pulp side. Place the potatoes with the skin side down on the baking sheet. Bake for 15 to 20 minutes, or until lightly browned.

Meanwhile, in a food processor or blender, process the remaining ingredients except the olives until smooth. Spoon about 1 teaspoon of the mixture into each baked potato skin. Top each piece with an olive slice.

....

COOK'S TIP: Save the potato pulp and use it to make mashed potatoes, shepherd's pie, or Chicken Pot Pie with Mashed Potato Topping (page 172). You can also use leftover potato pulp to thicken soups. The starch adds body. Puree the pulp with a small amount of broth for moisture and then stir the mixture into the soup.

....

COOK'S TIP: If you're in a hurry, you can "bake" the potatoes in the microwave. Using a fork, pierce each potato in several places. Wrap each in a paper towel. Place on a large microwaveable plate. Microwave on 100 percent power (high) for 10 minutes, or until the tines of a fork inserted into each potato come out easily. Remove from the microwave.

PER SERVING

Calories 54	Cholesterol 1 mg	DIETARY EXCHANGES:
Total Fat 0.5 g	Sodium 128 mg	½ starch
Saturated Fat 0.0 g	Carbohydrates 9 g	½ lean meat
Trans Fat 0.0 g	Fiber 1 g	
Polyunsaturated Fat 0.0 g	Sugars 2 g	
Monounsaturated Fat 0.0 g	Protein 4 g	

Kale-and-Ham-Stuffed Cremini Mushrooms

Serves 6

Kale gets sophisticated when it's used as part of a savory stuffing for cremini mushroom caps, which are then baked to create this elegant hors d'oeuvre.

- 1 tablespoon olive oil
- 1 medium onion, minced
- 2 medium garlic cloves, minced
- 12 large brown (cremini) mushrooms (about 14 ounces), stems removed and chopped
- 2 cups baby kale, coarsely chopped
- 3 ounces minced lower-sodium, low-fat ham, all visible fat discarded
- 1 cup whole-wheat panko (Japanese-style bread crumbs)
- 1 cup fat-free, low-sodium vegetable broth and ½ cup fat-free, low-sodium vegetable broth, divided use
- 2 tablespoons finely shredded or grated Parmesan cheese

Preheat the oven to 350°F.

In a large nonstick skillet, heat the oil over medium-high heat, swirling to coat the bottom. Cook the onion and garlic for about 2 minutes, or until the onion is almost soft, stirring frequently. Stir in the chopped mushroom stems, kale, and ham. Cook for 3 minutes, or until the mushrooms are soft, stirring occasionally. Stir in the panko and 1 cup broth. Cook for 3 to 5 minutes, or until heated through, stirring occasionally.

Stuff the mushroom caps with the kale mixture. Place on a rimmed baking sheet. Pour the remaining ½ cup broth over the mushrooms. Cover with aluminum foil.

Bake for 20 to 30 minutes, or until the mushroom caps are soft. Just before serving, sprinkle with the Parmesan.

PER SERVING

Calories 125	Cholesterol 7 mg	DIETARY EXCHANGES:
Total Fat 4.0 g	Sodium 180 mg	½ starch
Saturated Fat 1.0 g	Carbohydrates 17 g	1 vegetable
Trans Fat 0.0 g	Fiber 3 g	½ lean meat
Polyunsaturated Fat 0.5 g	Sugars 3 g	½ fat
Monounsaturated Fat 2.0 g	Protein 9 g	

Banana Mini Snack Cakes

Serves 12

Three fruits contribute flavor and moistness to these tiny snack cakes. Bake a batch to have handy for quick 100-calorie snacks, to pack in lunch boxes, and to grab when you're on the run.

> **Cooking spray**
> 1½ **cups white whole-wheat flour**
> ⅓ **cup firmly packed light brown sugar**
> 2 **teaspoons baking powder**
> ½ **teaspoon ground cinnamon**
> ¼ **teaspoon baking soda**
> ⅛ **teaspoon salt**
> ½ **cup mashed banana (about 1 medium)**
> ½ **cup fresh orange juice**
> ¼ **cup egg substitute**
> ¼ **cup unsweetened applesauce or 1 cup diced hulled strawberries**
> 1 **tablespoon canola or corn oil**
> 2 **teaspoons poppy seeds**

Preheat the oven to 400°F. Lightly spray one 12-cavity snack-cake pan, one standard 12-cup muffin pan, one 24-cup mini-muffin pan, or two 12-cup mini-muffin pans with cooking spray.

In a medium bowl, stir together the flour, brown sugar, baking powder, cinnamon, baking soda, and salt. In a separate medium bowl, stir together the remaining ingredients. Stir the banana mixture into the flour mixture until the batter is just moistened but no flour is visible. Don't overmix; the batter will be slightly lumpy. Spoon it into the pan.

Bake on the middle oven rack for 12 to 13 minutes, or until a wooden toothpick inserted in the center of a cake comes out clean.

Transfer the pan to a cooling rack and let cool for 5 minutes. Serve warm or at room temperature. Refrigerate any remaining cakes in an airtight plastic bag for up to five days or freeze for up to two months.

PER SERVING

Calories 105	Cholesterol 0 mg	DIETARY EXCHANGES:
Total Fat 2.0 g	Sodium 130 mg	1 starch
Saturated Fat 0.0 g	Carbohydrates 21 g	½ fruit
Trans Fat 0.0 g	Fiber 2 g	
Polyunsaturated Fat 0.5 g	Sugars 9 g	
Monounsaturated Fat 1.0 g	Protein 3 g	

Sangría-Style Pomegranate Coolers

Serves 6

Jewel-toned blueberry-pomegranate juice blends delightfully with zingy citrus juices to make this refreshing drink.

- 2 cups 100% blueberry-pomegranate juice or 100% pomegranate juice
- 2 medium limes, quartered
- 1 medium orange, cut into 8 wedges
- 2 cups diet ginger ale or Champagne (regular or nonalcoholic), chilled

Pour the pomegranate juice into a medium pitcher. Squeeze the juice of the limes and orange into the pitcher. Stir in the squeezed rinds. Cover with plastic wrap and refrigerate until chilled. (For a more pronounced citrus flavor, refrigerate for up to 24 hours.)

Just before serving, stir in the ginger ale. Serve with or without ice.

COOK'S TIP: Look in the produce section of your supermarket for 100% pomegranate juice bottled alone or combined with other 100% fruit juices.

PER SERVING

Calories 57	Cholesterol 0 mg	DIETARY EXCHANGES:
Total Fat 0.0 g	Sodium 30 mg	1 fruit
Saturated Fat 0.0 g	Carbohydrates 14 g	
Trans Fat 0.0 g	Fiber 0 g	
Polyunsaturated Fat 0.0 g	Sugars 13 g	
Monounsaturated Fat 0.0 g	Protein 1 g	

Orange-Strawberry Froth

Serves 6

Make your morning OJ a little more interesting with this fruity combo that takes no time at all to whip up as part of a healthy breakfast.

> 2 cups fresh orange juice
> 1½ cups 100% apricot nectar
> 1 cup frozen unsweetened strawberries

In a food processor or blender, process all the ingredients for 20 seconds, or until smooth and frothy. Serve immediately.

....

COOK'S TIP ON FRUIT NECTAR: Look for various fruit nectars in the juice section of your supermarket. Experiment with different kinds in this recipe for invigorating flavor changes.

....

PER SERVING

Calories 81	Cholesterol 0 mg	DIETARY EXCHANGES:
Total Fat 0.0 g	Sodium 3 mg	1½ fruit
Saturated Fat 0.0 g	Carbohydrates 20 g	
Trans Fat 0.0 g	Fiber 1 g	
Polyunsaturated Fat 0.0 g	Sugars 16 g	
Monounsaturated Fat 0.0 g	Protein 1 g	

Pineapple Shake

Serves 4

Forget those calorie-laden, sugar-loaded fast-food shakes and give this one a try. A tropical fruit adds natural sweetness to this super-simple shake, which takes less time than a trip through the drive-through.

1 **15.5-ounce can crushed pineapple in its own juice**
2 **cups fat-free, sugar-free frozen vanilla ice cream or yogurt**
1 **teaspoon vanilla extract**

In a food processor or blender, process all the ingredients until smooth.

PER SERVING

Calories 151	Cholesterol 0 mg	DIETARY EXCHANGES:
Total Fat 0.0 g	Sodium 59 mg	1 fruit
Saturated Fat 0.0 g	Carbohydrates 34 g	1½ other carbohydrate
Trans Fat 0.0 g	Fiber 1 g	
Polyunsaturated Fat 0.0 g	Sugars 18 g	
Monounsaturated Fat 0.0 g	Protein 3 g	

Spiced Apple Cider

Serves 16

A warm fire. A cozy room. A comfy chair. This cold-weather favorite completes the scene, without the added sugar found in many store-bought ciders.

- 2 quarts 100% apple juice or apple cider
- 1 quart water
- ½ medium orange, thinly sliced
- ½ medium lemon, thinly sliced
- 2 cinnamon sticks (each about 3 inches long)
- 12 whole allspice and ground allspice to taste, divided use
- 6 whole cloves
- 3 single-serving bags of unflavored tea (with a tag preferred)
  . . . .
- 1 medium orange, thinly sliced (optional)
- 1 medium lemon, thinly sliced (optional)

In a large stainless steel, enameled steel, or nonstick saucepan, bring the apple juice, water, slices of ½ orange and ½ lemon, cinnamon sticks, whole allspice, and cloves to a boil over high heat. Put the tea bags in the liquid, letting the tags hang over the side of the pan. Reduce the heat and simmer for 3 minutes. Discard the tea bags, orange and lemon slices, cinnamon sticks, whole allspice, and cloves. Simmer the liquid for 5 minutes.

Stir in the ground allspice.

Serve hot or cover and refrigerate to serve chilled. Garnish with the remaining orange and lemon slices.

COOK'S TIP ON BOUQUET GARNI: For easy removal of the whole allspice and cloves from the cider mixture, make a bouquet garni. Tie the spices in cheesecloth or put them in a large tea ball. When the cider is ready, you won't have to round up the spices, piece by piece. Most often made of parsley, thyme, and bay leaf, bouquets garnis are time-savers in soups and stews also.

PER SERVING

Calories 58	Cholesterol 0 mg	DIETARY EXCHANGES:
Total Fat 0.0 g	Sodium 7 mg	1 fruit
Saturated Fat 0.0 g	Carbohydrates 14 g	
Trans Fat 0.0 g	Fiber 0 g	
Polyunsaturated Fat 0.0 g	Sugars 12 g	
Monounsaturated Fat 0.0 g	Protein 0 g	

Soups

LIGHT AND LEMONY SPINACH SOUP 52

SILKY WINTER-SQUASH SOUP 53

CHUNKY BARLEY SOUP 54

COUNTRY-STYLE VEGETABLE SOUP 55

SUMMERTIME SOUP 56

PASTA-PARMESAN SOUP 57

CHILLED ASPARAGUS SOUP 58

GUMBO WITH GREENS AND HAM 60

BROCCOLI-CHEESE SOUP 62

CREAMY WILD RICE AND WHEAT BERRY SOUP 63

HOT-AND-SOUR SOUP WITH EXOTIC MUSHROOMS 64

RUSTIC TOMATO SOUP 66

SPICY CHICKPEA AND CHAYOTE SOUP 68

TRIPLE-PEPPER AND WHITE BEAN SOUP WITH ROTINI 69

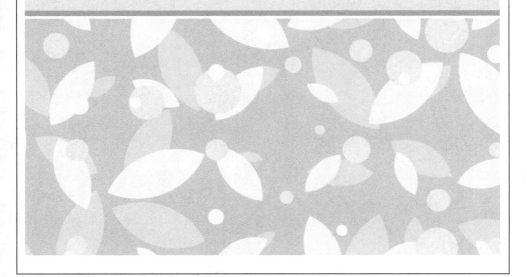

Light and Lemony Spinach Soup

Serves 2

This sunny soup takes just minutes to prepare, and you probably already have most of the ingredients in your kitchen. Try it with Mediterranean Grilled Salmon (page 123) and a side of steamed or sautéed spinach.

2 cups fat-free, low-sodium chicken broth
2 teaspoons fresh lemon juice
¼ teaspoon dried thyme, crumbled
¹⁄₁₆ teaspoon salt
4 spinach or other green leaves, such as kale or escarole, torn into bite-size pieces
1 medium green onion (green part only), thinly sliced

In a small saucepan, bring the broth, lemon juice, thyme, and salt to a boil over high heat.

Put the spinach in bowls. Ladle the soup over the spinach. Sprinkle with the green onion.

PER SERVING

Calories 21	Cholesterol 0 mg	DIETARY EXCHANGES:
Total Fat 0.0 g	Sodium 224 mg	Free
Saturated Fat 0.0 g	Carbohydrates 2 g	
Trans Fat 0.0 g	Fiber 1 g	
Polyunsaturated Fat 0.0 g	Sugars 1 g	
Monounsaturated Fat 0.0 g	Protein 3 g	

Silky Winter-Squash Soup

This creamy soup is sure to become a family favorite this fall. Roasting the vegetables intensifies their flavors and caramelizes their natural sugars.

Olive oil cooking spray

1 1-pound acorn squash, halved vertically, seeds and strings discarded

1 medium onion, halved

2 medium ribs of celery, cut into 2-inch pieces

½ cup baby carrots

4 medium garlic cloves, unpeeled

1 cup fat-free, low-sodium chicken broth and 2 cups fat-free, low-sodium chicken broth, divided use

¼ cup fat-free half-and-half

¼ teaspoon ground cumin

¼ teaspoon pepper

⅛ teaspoon salt

Preheat the oven to 350°F. Lightly spray a 13 x 9 x 2-inch baking dish with cooking spray.

Put the squash and onion with the cut sides up in the baking dish. Place the celery and carrots around the squash and onion. Lightly spray the vegetables with cooking spray. Bake for 45 minutes, or until the vegetables are just past tender-crisp. Add the garlic. Bake for 15 minutes, or until the vegetables are tender when pierced with the tip of a sharp knife. Transfer the baking dish to a cooling rack. Let cool for 10 minutes.

Using a spoon, scoop the pulp from the squash. Peel the garlic, discarding the skin. In a food processor or blender, process the pulp, onion, celery, carrots, garlic, and 1 cup broth for 1 to 2 minutes, or until smooth, scraping the side as necessary. Transfer to a medium saucepan.

Stir in the remaining ingredients, including the remaining 2 cups broth. Bring to a simmer over medium-high heat, stirring occasionally. Reduce the heat and simmer for 5 to 6 minutes, stirring occasionally.

PER SERVING

Calories 79	Cholesterol 0 mg	DIETARY EXCHANGES:
Total Fat 0.5 g	Sodium 160 mg	1 starch
Saturated Fat 0.0 g	Carbohydrates 17 g	1 vegetable
Trans Fat 0.0 g	Fiber 3 g	
Polyunsaturated Fat 0.0 g	Sugars 6 g	
Monounsaturated Fat 0.0 g	Protein 4 g	

Chunky Barley Soup

Serves 4

Cumin adds just a hint of smokiness to this robust side soup complete with a whole grain and vegetables.

¼ cup fat-free sour cream
½ teaspoon bottled white horseradish, drained
⅛ teaspoon dried basil, crumbled
1 teaspoon olive oil
1 medium rib of celery, chopped
½ medium onion, chopped
½ medium red bell pepper, chopped
½ cup frozen whole-kernel corn, thawed
½ teaspoon ground cumin
¼ teaspoon pepper
⅛ teaspoon salt
3½ cups fat-free, low-sodium chicken broth
⅓ cup uncooked quick-cooking barley

In a small bowl, whisk together the sour cream, horseradish, and basil. Cover and refrigerate until serving time.

In a medium saucepan, heat the oil over medium-high heat, swirling to coat the bottom. Cook the celery, onion, and bell pepper for 3 to 4 minutes, or until the onion is soft, stirring frequently.

Stir in the corn, cumin, pepper, and salt. Cook for 1 minute, or until the cumin is fragrant.

Stir in the broth and barley. Bring to a simmer. Reduce the heat and simmer, covered, for 10 minutes, or until the barley is tender.

Just before serving, garnish with the sour cream mixture.

PER SERVING

Calories 126	Cholesterol 3 mg	DIETARY EXCHANGES:
Total Fat 1.5 g	Sodium 153 mg	1½ starch
Saturated Fat 0.0 g	Carbohydrates 23 g	
Trans Fat 0.0 g	Fiber 4 g	
Polyunsaturated Fat 0.5 g	Sugars 4 g	
Monounsaturated Fat 1.0 g	Protein 6 g	

Country-Style Vegetable Soup

Serves 10

The variety of fresh vegetables in this hearty side soup makes it a perfect complement to any entrée. Try it with Crispy Oven-Fried Chicken (page 144) or Ham and Rice Croquettes (page 204).

  1 **pound white or red potatoes, chopped**
  4 **large carrots, chopped**
  3 **medium ribs of celery with leaves, chopped**
  2 **medium zucchini, chopped**
  1 **medium onion, chopped**
  ¼ **cup chopped fresh parsley**
  2 **medium dried bay leaves**
  ⅛ **teaspoon salt**
     Pepper to taste
  6 **cups fat-free, low-sodium chicken broth**
  ¾ **cup shredded low-fat Cheddar cheese**

In a large, heavy saucepan or Dutch oven, stir together the potatoes, carrots, celery, zucchini, onion, parsley, bay leaves, salt, and pepper.

Stir in the broth. Bring to a boil over high heat. Reduce the heat and simmer, covered, for 45 minutes to 1 hour, or until the vegetables are very tender. Discard the bay leaves.

Just before serving, sprinkle with the Cheddar.

. . . .

COOK'S TIP: If you want the celery to retain its crunch, don't add it until about 10 minutes before the soup is ready.

. . . .

PER SERVING

Calories 82	Cholesterol 2 mg	DIETARY EXCHANGES:
Total Fat 1.0 g	Sodium 153 mg	½ starch
Saturated Fat 0.5 g	Carbohydrates 14 g	1 vegetable
Trans Fat 0.0 g	Fiber 2 g	½ lean meat
Polyunsaturated Fat 0.0 g	Sugars 4 g	
Monounsaturated Fat 0.0 g	Protein 5 g	

Summertime Soup

When you've just stocked up on fresh summer fruits from the farmers' market, try this refreshing cold soup to enjoy their natural flavors in a whole new way.

SOUP

1	small cantaloupe, cubed
2	large mangoes, cubed
2	medium peaches, peeled and cubed
16	ounces strawberries, hulled
½	cup fat-free plain Greek yogurt
⅓	cup frozen 100% orange juice concentrate, slightly thawed
⅓	cup port wine or 100% grape juice
2	tablespoons orange liqueur (optional)
1	tablespoon fresh lime juice
1½	teaspoons raspberry vinegar

. . . .

½	cup fat-free plain Greek yogurt

In a food processor or blender, process all the soup ingredients until thick and creamy. Pour into a large bowl. Cover and put in the freezer for about 20 minutes.

Just before serving, remove the soup from the freezer. Dollop with the remaining ½ cup yogurt.

PER SERVING

Calories 221	Cholesterol 0 mg	DIETARY EXCHANGES:
Total Fat 1.0 g	Sodium 30 mg	3 fruit
Saturated Fat 0.0 g	Carbohydrates 47 g	1 lean meat
Trans Fat 0.0 g	Fiber 5 g	
Polyunsaturated Fat 0.5 g	Sugars 21 g	
Monounsaturated Fat 0.5 g	Protein 7 g	

Pasta-Parmesan Soup

Serves 6

Light but filling, this soup is good year-round and can be made anytime because it uses ingredients you probably have on hand. Add leftover diced chicken breast to turn this easy appetizer into an entrée.

½ **cup egg substitute**

4 **cups fat-free, low-sodium chicken broth**

1 **cup dried whole-grain pastina or any crushed dried whole-grain macaroni**

¼ **cup shredded or grated Parmesan cheese**

1 **tablespoon chopped fresh parsley**

In a small bowl, whisk the egg substitute until thoroughly blended.

In a medium saucepan, bring the broth to a simmer over medium heat. Stir in the pasta. Return the broth to a simmer. Reduce the heat and simmer for 10 minutes, or until the pasta is tender, stirring occasionally.

Whisk in the egg substitute. Cook for 1 minute. Just before serving, sprinkle with the Parmesan and parsley.

PER SERVING

Calories 93	Cholesterol 2 mg	DIETARY EXCHANGES:
Total Fat 1.5 g	Sodium 115 mg	1 starch
Saturated Fat 0.5 g	Carbohydrates 14 g	½ lean meat
Trans Fat 0.0 g	Fiber 2 g	
Polyunsaturated Fat 0.0 g	Sugars 1 g	
Monounsaturated Fat 0.5 g	Protein 7 g	

Chilled Asparagus Soup

Serves 4

Try this cool make-ahead soup in spring and summer, when fresh asparagus is plentiful. This soup's mild seasoning makes it a perfect starter for nearly any meal. If you'd like a vegetarian version, use fat-free, low-sodium vegetable broth.

2 cups asparagus spears, trimmed and cut into ¾-inch pieces (about 8 ounces)
1½ cups fat-free, low-sodium chicken broth and ½ cup fat-free, low-sodium chicken broth, divided use
½ cup chopped onion
1 to 2 teaspoons grated peeled gingerroot
1 tablespoon cornstarch
⅛ teaspoon salt
⅓ cup fat-free sour cream

In a medium saucepan, stir together the asparagus, 1½ cups broth, the onion, and gingerroot. Bring to a boil over medium-high heat. Reduce the heat and simmer, covered, for about 5 minutes, or until the asparagus is tender and the onion is soft.

In a food processor or blender (vent the blender lid), process half the soup until smooth. Carefully return the pureed soup to the pan.

Put the cornstarch in a small bowl. Add the remaining ½ cup broth, whisking to dissolve. Whisk into the soup. Whisk in the salt. Cook for 4 minutes, or until the soup has thickened, whisking constantly.

Transfer the soup to a large serving bowl. Cover and refrigerate for at least 2 hours, or until chilled. Just before serving, whisk in the sour cream.

COOK'S TIP ON BLENDING HOT LIQUIDS: Be careful when blending hot liquids. Venting the blender lid prevents heat and steam from popping off the lid. Most blender lids have a center section that can be removed. You can even place a kitchen towel over the opening to avoid splatters. Begin blending at the lowest speed and increase to the desired speed, holding the lid down firmly.

COOK'S TIP ON ASPARAGUS: An asparagus spear has a natural bending point where the tough stem ends. Holding a spear at the top and bottom, bend the spear; snap at the bending point. Discard the tough stem or reserve it to use in making broth or other soups.

PER SERVING

Calories 55
Total Fat 0.0 g
  Saturated Fat 0.0 g
  Trans Fat 0.0 g
  Polyunsaturated Fat 0.0 g
  Monounsaturated Fat 0.0 g

Cholesterol 3 mg
Sodium 105 mg
Carbohydrates 10 g
  Fiber 2 g
  Sugars 4 g
Protein 4 g

DIETARY EXCHANGES:
1 vegetable
½ starch

Gumbo with Greens and Ham

Serves 8

Browning the flour adds a depth of flavor to this gumbo without the extra fat of a roux. The "holy trinity" of onion, celery, and bell pepper—along with okra and fresh greens—gives this entrée soup an authentic Cajun taste.

½ cup all-purpose flour
1¼ cups uncooked brown rice
   Cooking spray
2 medium onions, chopped
2 medium ribs of celery, chopped
1 medium yellow or green bell pepper, chopped
1 medium red bell pepper, chopped
6 medium garlic cloves, minced
3 cups water
2 cups chopped lower-sodium, low-fat ham, all visible fat discarded
1½ cups sliced fresh or frozen okra, thawed if frozen
6 ounces collard greens, mustard greens, kale, or spinach, coarsely chopped
2 bunches of watercress, coarsely chopped
1 bunch of fresh parsley, coarsely chopped
¼ to ½ teaspoon pepper
¼ teaspoon red hot-pepper sauce, or to taste
⅛ to ¼ teaspoon cayenne

Heat a large, heavy saucepan or Dutch oven over medium-high heat. Cook the flour for 5 minutes, stirring occasionally. Reduce the heat to medium and cook for 5 to 7 minutes, or until evenly browned, stirring constantly. Transfer to a small bowl or plate. Allow the pan to cool.

Prepare the rice using the package directions, omitting the salt and margarine.

Meanwhile, lightly spray the cooled pan with cooking spray. Cook the onions, celery, bell peppers, and garlic over medium heat for 15 minutes, stirring occasionally.

Stir in the browned flour and the remaining ingredients except the rice. Increase the heat to high and bring to a boil. Reduce the heat and simmer, covered, for 30 minutes.

Spoon the rice into bowls. Ladle the gumbo over the rice.

PER SERVING

Calories 217	Cholesterol 15 mg	DIETARY EXCHANGES:
Total Fat 2.5 g	Sodium 346 mg	2 starch
Saturated Fat 0.5 g	Carbohydrates 39 g	2 vegetable
Trans Fat 0.0 g	Fiber 4 g	1 lean meat
Polyunsaturated Fat 0.5 g	Sugars 5 g	
Monounsaturated Fat 1.0 g	Protein 11 g	

Broccoli-Cheese Soup

Serves 4

This entrée soup has all the creaminess you expect, but with less saturated fat and sodium. Serve it with a crusty whole-grain roll.

- 2½ cups fat-free, low-sodium chicken broth
- 6 ounces chopped broccoli or 10 ounces frozen chopped broccoli, thawed
- 1 medium carrot, chopped
- 1 medium rib of celery, chopped
- ¼ teaspoon salt
- ¼ teaspoon pepper
- ⅛ teaspoon ground nutmeg
- 3 tablespoons all-purpose flour
- 1 cup fat-free half-and-half
- 3 slices (about ¾ ounce each) low-fat sharp Cheddar cheese, torn into pieces, or ½ cup shredded low-fat sharp Cheddar cheese

In a large saucepan, stir together the broth, broccoli, carrot, celery, salt, pepper, and nutmeg. Bring to a simmer over medium-high heat. Reduce the heat and simmer, covered, for 6 to 8 minutes, or until the vegetables are tender.

Put the flour in a small bowl. Pour in the half-and-half, whisking until smooth. Whisk the mixture into the soup. Simmer for 1 to 2 minutes, or until the soup is thickened, stirring occasionally.

Add the Cheddar. Remove from the heat.

Stir the soup until the Cheddar is melted.

....

COOK'S TIP: One of the best ways to reheat this soup and keep it from being scorched is to use a double boiler. Pour the soup into the top pan of the double boiler and heat over simmering water. If you don't have a double boiler, place a medium stainless steel bowl over a pan of simmering water. In either case, be sure the water in the bottom pan doesn't touch the top container.

....

PER SERVING

Calories 119	Cholesterol 3 mg	DIETARY EXCHANGES:
Total Fat 1.5 g	Sodium 375 mg	1 starch
Saturated Fat 0.5 g	Carbohydrates 18 g	1 vegetable
Trans Fat 0.0 g	Fiber 2 g	1 lean meat
Polyunsaturated Fat 0.0 g	Sugars 6 g	
Monounsaturated Fat 0.5 g	Protein 11 g	

Creamy Wild Rice and Wheat Berry Soup

Serves 4

Adding a variety of whole grains to your diet is easier than you may think. This soup provides two: wild rice (actually the seed of an annual marsh grass, but it counts as a grain) and wheat berries.

- 2 cups water
- 1 cup fat-free, low-sodium chicken broth
- 1 large onion, chopped
- 2 medium ribs of celery, chopped
- ¼ cup wild rice, rinsed and drained
- ¼ cup wheat berries, rinsed and drained
- 2 medium garlic cloves, minced
- ½ teaspoon curry powder
- ¼ teaspoon pepper
- 1 12-ounce can fat-free evaporated milk
- 2 tablespoons dry sherry (optional)
- 4 very thin lemon slices (optional)
- 2 tablespoons chopped fresh parsley (optional)

In a large saucepan, stir together the water, broth, onion, celery, rice, wheat berries, garlic, curry powder, and pepper. Bring to a boil over high heat. Reduce the heat and simmer, covered, for 1 hour, or until the rice is tender.

Stir in the milk and sherry. Simmer until heated through.

Just before serving, garnish with the lemon and parsley.

....

COOK'S TIP ON WHEAT BERRIES: Nutty-tasting, chewy wheat berries are wheat kernels without the inedible outer hulls. Look for this nutritious grain in health food stores and some supermarkets. If you can't find wheat berries, use one-half cup of wild rice instead of one-quarter cup.

....

PER SERVING

Calories 173	Cholesterol 3 mg	DIETARY EXCHANGES:
Total Fat 0.5 g	Sodium 136 mg	1 starch
Saturated Fat 0.0 g	Carbohydrates 33 g	1 fat-free milk
Trans Fat 0.0 g	Fiber 4 g	1 vegetable
Polyunsaturated Fat 0.0 g	Sugars 13 g	
Monounsaturated Fat 0.0 g	Protein 11 g	

Hot-and-Sour Soup with Exotic Mushrooms

Serves 8

Make the most of the variety of fresh mushrooms available at your local market with this tangy, peppery soup. Strips of lean pork add meatiness, while snow peas and water chestnuts provide crunch.

4	cups fat-free, low-sodium chicken broth
1	pound mixed mushrooms, such as cremini (brown), enoki, oyster, portobello, shiitake (stems discarded), wood ear, and button, larger mushrooms cut into ¼-inch slices
2	boneless center-cut pork chops (about 4 ounces each), all visible fat discarded, cut into 2 x ¼-inch strips
¼	cup cider vinegar
1½	tablespoons soy sauce (lowest sodium available)
2	teaspoons toasted sesame oil
1	teaspoon sugar
¼ to ½	teaspoon pepper (white preferred)
3	tablespoons cornstarch
¼	cup water
1	8-ounce can sliced water chestnuts, drained
6	ounces snow peas, trimmed
¼	cup egg substitute, lightly beaten

In a large saucepan, bring the broth, mushrooms, pork, vinegar, soy sauce, sesame oil, sugar, and pepper to a boil over high heat, stirring occasionally. Reduce the heat and simmer for 10 minutes, or until the mushrooms are soft and the pork is no longer pink in the center, stirring occasionally.

Put the cornstarch in a small bowl. Add the water, whisking to dissolve. Stir into the soup. Increase the heat to medium high and cook for 2 to 3 minutes, or until the soup is thickened, stirring occasionally.

Stir in the water chestnuts and peas. Cook for 1 to 2 minutes, or until the peas are tender-crisp, stirring occasionally.

Slowly drizzle the egg substitute into the soup. Cook for 1 minute, or until the ribbons of egg substitute are cooked through, stirring constantly but gently. Serve immediately.

COOK'S TIP ON DRIED MUSHROOMS: Can't find your favorite fresh mushroom? Feel free to substitute dried mushrooms. Cover them with warm water and soak them for 20 to 30 minutes, or until softened. Drain them, squeezing out any excess water, and proceed with the recipe. Keep in mind that 1 ounce of dried mushrooms equals about 1 cup of rehydrated mushrooms.

COOK'S TIP ON SESAME OIL: Toasted sesame oil, also called Asian sesame oil, is darker, stronger, and more fragrant than other sesame oils. Toasted sesame oil is widely used in Asian and Indian foods. Because its flavor is so intense, you can use just a little for lots of taste and spare yourself some fat.

PER SERVING

Calories 103	Cholesterol 15 mg	DIETARY EXCHANGES:
Total Fat 3.0 g	Sodium 139 mg	2 vegetable
Saturated Fat 0.5 g	Carbohydrates 10 g	1 lean meat
Trans Fat 0.0 g	Fiber 2 g	
Polyunsaturated Fat 1.0 g	Sugars 3 g	
Monounsaturated Fat 1.0 g	Protein 10 g	

Rustic Tomato Soup

Serves 6

This classic sandwich partner can stand on its own, with its filling addition of pasta and chickpeas, but a smaller portion of it also pairs well with a low-fat grilled cheese sandwich (go ahead and dunk it; we won't tell!).

1   teaspoon olive oil
1   small onion, chopped
1   medium rib of celery, chopped
2   medium garlic cloves, minced
2   cups water
1   14.5-ounce can no-salt-added diced tomatoes, undrained
1   8-ounce can no-salt-added tomato sauce
1½ tablespoons Worcestershire sauce (lowest sodium available)
2   packets (2 teaspoons) salt-free instant chicken bouillon
2   teaspoons sugar
1½ teaspoons dried oregano, crumbled
½   teaspoon dried basil, crumbled
½   teaspoon pepper
⅔   cup dried whole-grain elbow macaroni
1   15.5-ounce can no-salt-added chickpeas or cannellini beans, rinsed and drained
½   cup fat-free half-and-half
2   tablespoons shredded or grated Parmesan cheese

In a medium saucepan, heat the oil over medium-high heat, swirling to coat the bottom. Cook the onion and celery for 3 minutes, or until soft, stirring occasionally. Stir in the garlic. Cook for 30 seconds, stirring frequently.

In a food processor or blender, process the onion mixture, water, tomatoes with liquid, tomato sauce, and Worcestershire sauce for about 20 seconds, or until almost smooth, scraping the side once with a rubber scraper. Return the mixture to the pan.

Stir in the bouillon, sugar, oregano, basil, and pepper. Bring to a boil, still over medium-high heat.

Stir in the pasta. Reduce the heat and simmer for 8 to 10 minutes, or until the pasta is tender, stirring occasionally.

Stir in the chickpeas. Cook for 1 minute, or until heated through. Remove from the heat.

Stir in the half-and-half. Just before serving, sprinkle with the Parmesan.

PER SERVING

Calories 173	Cholesterol 1 mg	DIETARY EXCHANGES:
Total Fat 2.0 g	Sodium 129 mg	1½ starch
Saturated Fat 0.5 g	Carbohydrates 32 g	2 vegetable
Trans Fat 0.0 g	Fiber 6 g	
Polyunsaturated Fat 0.0 g	Sugars 10 g	
Monounsaturated Fat 0.5 g	Protein 9 g	

Spicy Chickpea and Chayote Soup

Serves 4

Chayote squash is a mildly flavored summer squash often used in Mexican and Central American cooking. Pair this vegetarian entrée with a salad of dark, leafy greens and a whole-grain roll for a delicious lunch or light dinner.

1	medium chayote squash, peeled, pitted, and diced
2¼	cups no-salt-added tomato juice
3	tablespoons no-salt-added tomato paste
2	medium garlic cloves, minced, or 1 teaspoon bottled minced garlic
¼ to ½	teaspoon red hot-pepper sauce, or to taste
1	15.5-ounce can no-salt-added chickpeas, rinsed and drained
¾	cup cubed cooked skinless chicken or turkey breast, cooked without salt, all visible fat discarded
½	teaspoon dried oregano, crumbled
¼	teaspoon salt
¼	teaspoon pepper (white preferred)
2	tablespoons chopped fresh cilantro or parsley

Put the squash in a small saucepan. Pour in enough water to cover it by 1 inch. Bring to a boil over high heat. Boil for 8 to 10 minutes, or until tender, stirring occasionally. Drain well in a colander.

Meanwhile, in a large saucepan, stir together the tomato juice, tomato paste, garlic, and hot-pepper sauce. Cook over medium-high heat for 4 to 5 minutes, stirring occasionally.

Stir in the squash and the remaining ingredients except the cilantro. Reduce the heat and simmer, partially covered, for 5 minutes. Just before serving, sprinkle with the cilantro.

PER SERVING

Calories 209	Cholesterol 22 mg	DIETARY EXCHANGES:
Total Fat 2.5 g	Sodium 298 mg	1½ starch
Saturated Fat 0.5 g	Carbohydrates 31 g	2 vegetable
Trans Fat 0.0 g	Fiber 7 g	1½ lean meat
Polyunsaturated Fat 0.5 g	Sugars 9 g	
Monounsaturated Fat 0.5 g	Protein 16 g	

Triple-Pepper and White Bean Soup with Rotini

Serves 4

This vegetarian meal in a bowl is rich in protein and fiber, thanks to the addition of navy beans and whole-grain pasta. Tomatoes and zucchini add color, while a frozen mix of bell peppers and onion keeps prep time to a minimum.

2 cups fat-free, low-sodium vegetable broth

8 ounces frozen red and green bell pepper and onion stir-fry mixture

1 medium zucchini, halved lengthwise, then sliced crosswise

1 cup quartered cherry tomatoes

1 tablespoon dried basil, crumbled

⅛ teaspoon crushed red pepper flakes

6 ounces dried whole-grain rotini

1 15.5-ounce can no-salt-added navy beans, rinsed and drained

1 tablespoon olive oil (extra virgin preferred)

¼ teaspoon salt

In a large, heavy saucepan or Dutch oven, bring the broth to a boil over high heat. Stir in the stir-fry mix, zucchini, tomatoes, basil, and red pepper flakes. Return to a boil. Reduce the heat and simmer, covered, for 20 minutes.

Meanwhile, prepare the pasta using the package directions, omitting the salt. Drain well in a colander.

Stir the beans into the soup. Cook for 5 minutes, or until heated through. Remove from the heat.

Stir in the oil and salt.

Spoon the pasta into bowls. Ladle the soup over the pasta.

PER SERVING

Calories 313	Cholesterol 0 mg	DIETARY EXCHANGES:
Total Fat 4.5 g	Sodium 174 mg	3 starch
Saturated Fat 0.5 g	Carbohydrates 58 g	2 vegetable
Trans Fat 0.0 g	Fiber 10 g	½ lean meat
Polyunsaturated Fat 0.5 g	Sugars 9 g	
Monounsaturated Fat 2.5 g	Protein 14 g	

Salads and Salad Dressings

BOSTON CITRUS SALAD 72

FENNEL-ORANGE SALAD 74

CUCUMBER-MELON
SALAD WITH RASPBERRY
VINEGAR 75

GREEN BEAN AND TOASTED
PECAN SALAD 76

WARM MUSHROOM SALAD 77

ASIAN-STYLE SLAW 78

JÍCAMA AND GRAPEFRUIT
SALAD WITH ANCHO-HONEY
DRESSING 80

CITRUS RICE SALAD 82

LEMON-CURRIED
BLACK-EYED PEA SALAD 84

TABBOULEH 86

SEAFOOD PASTA SALAD 88

HERBED CHICKEN SALAD 89

ROASTED POTATO AND
CHICKEN SALAD WITH GREEK
DRESSING 90

ARTICHOKE-ROTINI SALAD
WITH CHICKEN 92

GREEK CHOPPED SALAD 93

TACO SALAD 94

MACARONI SALAD WITH
RICOTTA 96

CREAMY ARTICHOKE
DRESSING 97

CREAMY HERB DRESSING 98

GAZPACHO DRESSING 99

PARMESAN-PEPPERCORN
RANCH DRESSING 100

TOMATILLO-AVOCADO
DRESSING 101

CITRUS-TARRAGON
VINAIGRETTE 102

Boston Citrus Salad

Serves 6

Delicate, pale-green Boston lettuce is the perfect backdrop for juicy citrus fruit. The orange-flower water lends an aromatic touch to this salad, but leave it out if you can't find it.

1	large head of Boston, butter, or Bibb lettuce, leaves torn into bite-size pieces
2	large oranges
2	medium grapefruit
1½	tablespoons fresh lemon juice
1½	tablespoons honey
½	teaspoon orange-flower water or orange liqueur (optional)
3	tablespoons slivered almonds, dry-roasted

Put the lettuce in a large bowl.

Peel the oranges. Cut crosswise into ¼-inch slices. Cut the slices into quarters. Transfer the oranges to a medium bowl and any accumulated juice to a small bowl.

Peel and section the grapefruit. Cut into bite-size pieces. Add the grapefruit to the oranges and any accumulated grapefruit juice to the orange juice. Drain the fruit, adding any accumulated juice to the juice mixture.

Stir the lemon juice, honey, and orange-flower water into the juice mixture. Pour over the lettuce, tossing to coat.

Arrange the lettuce on salad plates. Top each serving with the orange and grapefruit pieces. Sprinkle with the almonds.

....

COOK'S TIP ON GRAPEFRUIT: Grapefruit can interact with a number of medications, including many heart medicines. Be sure to check with your doctor or pharmacist if you take any medication, and use large oranges, pomelos, or another fruit as an alternate ingredient if necessary.

....

COOK'S TIP ON ORANGE-FLOWER WATER: Orange-flower water, found at Middle Eastern markets, most gourmet grocery stores, and some supermarkets, is a flavorful and fragrant addition to many cakes, cookies, puddings, and beverages.

PER SERVING

Calories 97	Cholesterol 0 mg	DIETARY EXCHANGES:
Total Fat 2.0 g	Sodium 2 mg	1½ fruit
Saturated Fat 0.0 g	Carbohydrates 20 g	½ fat
Trans Fat 0.0 g	Fiber 3 g	
Polyunsaturated Fat 0.5 g	Sugars 17 g	
Monounsaturated Fat 1.0 g	Protein 2 g	

Fennel-Orange Salad

The feathery tops of the mildly licorice-tasting fennel bulb help flavor the dressing that enhances this crisp salad, which blends bitter greens and sweet fruit.

DRESSING

- 3 tablespoons white wine vinegar
- 1 tablespoon olive oil (extra virgin preferred)
- 2 teaspoons honey
- 1 teaspoon chopped fennel fronds (optional)
- 1 medium garlic clove, minced
- ½ teaspoon grated orange zest
- ⅛ teaspoon salt
- ⅛ teaspoon pepper

SALAD

- 4 cups torn romaine
- 1 cup torn radicchio
- 2 medium fennel bulbs, ends trimmed, thinly sliced
- 2 medium oranges, peeled and cut crosswise into slices, seeds discarded

In a small bowl, whisk together the dressing ingredients.

In a large bowl, toss together the romaine and radicchio. Scatter the fennel on top. Pour the dressing over all, tossing gently to coat. Arrange the orange slices on the salad.

PER SERVING

Calories 123	Cholesterol 0 mg	DIETARY EXCHANGES:
Total Fat 4.0 g	Sodium 140 mg	1 fruit
Saturated Fat 0.5 g	Carbohydrates 22 g	2 vegetable
Trans Fat 0.0 g	Fiber 6 g	1 fat
Polyunsaturated Fat 0.5 g	Sugars 10 g	
Monounsaturated Fat 2.5 g	Protein 3 g	

74   **HEALTHY FATS, LOW-CHOLESTEROL COOKBOOK**

Cucumber-Melon Salad with Raspberry Vinegar

Serves 4

Expand your taste horizons by trying this unusual combination of mild, sweet, bitter, and tart ingredients. Omit the lettuce and finely chop the cucumber, cantaloupe, and radishes to create a cooling summer relish to serve with grilled fish, such as Grilled Cod with Artichoke-Horseradish Sauce (page 114).

> 1 medium cucumber, strips of peel removed from part of the cucumber (leave some dark green for color), cut into bite-size pieces
> 3 cups cantaloupe cubes
> 1 bunch of radishes, thinly sliced
> ¼ cup raspberry vinegar
> Pepper to taste (optional)
> 4 large lettuce leaves

In a medium bowl, stir together the cucumber, cantaloupe, radishes, and vinegar, tossing to coat.

Sprinkle with the pepper. Cover and refrigerate for 30 minutes to 1 hour, or until chilled.

Place the lettuce on salad plates. Spoon the salad over the lettuce.

. . . .

COOK'S TIP: You can also use a melon baller for the cantaloupe and scoop out small ball-size pieces if you prefer these to cubes.

. . . .

PER SERVING

Calories 53	Cholesterol 0 mg	DIETARY EXCHANGES:
Total Fat 0.5 g	Sodium 26 mg	1 fruit
Saturated Fat 0.0 g	Carbohydrates 12 g	
Trans Fat 0.0 g	Fiber 2 g	
Polyunsaturated Fat 0.0 g	Sugars 10 g	
Monounsaturated Fat 0.0 g	Protein 2 g	

Green Bean and Toasted Pecan Salad

Serves 4

Break away from standard lettuce salads or slaws. Try this picture-perfect veggie salad with its bright green beans and purple rings of red onion. It's no slouch in the taste category, either, thanks to tangy blue cheese and a sprinkling of crunchy pecans.

12 **ounces whole green beans, trimmed**
⅛ **to ¼ cup thinly sliced red onion**
1½ **tablespoons white balsamic vinegar**
2¼ **teaspoons sugar**
⅛ **teaspoon salt**
2 **tablespoons finely chopped pecans, dry-roasted**
2 **tablespoons crumbled low-fat blue cheese**

In a medium saucepan, steam the green beans for 4 minutes, or just until tender-crisp. Transfer to a colander and rinse with cold water to stop the cooking process. Let cool to room temperature. Drain well. Dry on paper towels.

Meanwhile, in a medium serving bowl, stir together the onion, vinegar, sugar, and salt.

Add the green beans, tossing to combine.

Sprinkle with the pecans and blue cheese.

PER SERVING

Calories 76	Cholesterol 2 mg	DIETARY EXCHANGES:
Total Fat 3.5 g	Sodium 127 mg	2 vegetable
Saturated Fat 0.5 g	Carbohydrates 11 g	½ fat
Trans Fat 0.0 g	Fiber 3 g	
Polyunsaturated Fat 1.0 g	Sugars 7 g	
Monounsaturated Fat 1.5 g	Protein 3 g	

Warm Mushroom Salad

Serves 4

Balsamic vinegar imparts a deep, rich flavor to mushrooms. If you wish, you can use meaty-textured portobello mushrooms and serve this salad as part of a meatless meal.

<ul>
<li>¼ cup port, sweet red wine (regular or nonalcoholic), or frozen 100% apple juice concentrate, thawed</li>
<li>3 to 3½ tablespoons balsamic vinegar or plain rice vinegar</li>
<li>2 tablespoons water</li>
<li>3 medium garlic cloves, finely minced</li>
<li>12 ounces button or portobello mushrooms, cut into ¼-inch slices</li>
<li>1 teaspoon olive oil (extra virgin preferred)</li>
<li>⅛ teaspoon pepper, or to taste</li>
<li>4 Boston lettuce leaves</li>
<li>1 teaspoon chopped fresh parsley</li>
</ul>

In a medium nonstick skillet, whisk together the port, vinegar, water, and garlic. Cook over medium-high heat until small bubbles begin to form.

Stir in the mushrooms. Cook for 8 to 10 minutes, or until all the liquid has evaporated, stirring frequently.

Stir in the oil and pepper.

Place the lettuce leaves on salad plates. Spoon the mushrooms over the lettuce. Sprinkle with the parsley. Serve immediately.

PER SERVING

Calories 68	Cholesterol 0 mg	DIETARY EXCHANGES:
Total Fat 1.5 g	Sodium 10 mg	½ other carbohydrate
Saturated Fat 0.0 g	Carbohydrates 9 g	½ fat
Trans Fat 0.0 g	Fiber 1 g	
Polyunsaturated Fat 0.5 g	Sugars 6 g	
Monounsaturated Fat 1.0 g	Protein 3 g	

Asian-Style Slaw

Serves 8

Topped with golden-brown, baked wonton strips that contribute extra crunch, this slaw makes an attractive presentation alongside Grilled Teriyaki Sirloin (page 182).

Cooking spray
8 **wonton wrappers**
¼ **teaspoon five-spice powder or salt-free all-purpose seasoning blend**
2 **tablespoons all-fruit apricot spread**
2 **tablespoons fresh orange juice**
1 **tablespoon cider vinegar**
2 **teaspoons canola or corn oil**
1 **teaspoon toasted sesame oil**
2 **cups shredded green cabbage**
1 **cup shredded red cabbage**
1 **medium carrot, shredded**
6 **medium radishes, thinly sliced**
2 **medium green onions, thinly sliced**

Preheat the oven to 400°F. Lightly spray a baking sheet with cooking spray.

Cut the wonton wrappers into strips ¼ inch wide. Arrange the strips in a single layer on the baking sheet (they don't have to be perfectly straight; a slight twist or bend looks interesting). Lightly spray the strips with cooking spray.

Sprinkle the five-spice powder over the strips. Bake for 5 to 6 minutes, or until golden brown. Transfer the baking sheet to a cooling rack and let the strips cool for 5 to 10 minutes.

In a medium bowl, whisk together the fruit spread, orange juice, vinegar, and both oils.

Stir in the remaining ingredients, tossing to coat.

Mound the slaw on salad plates. Sprinkle with the wonton strips.

....

COOK'S TIP: A package of wonton wrappers will provide more than you need for this recipe. Separate the extras into batches of eight so you'll be ready to make this slaw again, then freeze them in plastic freezer bags or other airtight containers for up to four months. You can also cut all the wrappers into strips and then bake them. Store them in an airtight container at room temperature for up to five days. Use them to top soups or salads.

....

COOK'S TIP ON FIVE-SPICE POWDER: You can usually find five-spice powder in the spice section of your grocery store and in Asian markets. If you prefer, you can easily make your own. Simply combine equal amounts of cinnamon, cloves, fennel seed, star anise, and Szechuan peppercorns, all in ground form. If Szechuan peppercorns aren't readily available, substitute black pepper; if you can't find star anise, the mixture will still provide plenty of flavor if you leave it out.

PER SERVING

Calories 65	Cholesterol 1 mg	DIETARY EXCHANGES:
Total Fat 2.0 g	Sodium 60 mg	½ starch
Saturated Fat 0.0 g	Carbohydrates 11 g	1 vegetable
Trans Fat 0.0 g	Fiber 1 g	
Polyunsaturated Fat 0.5 g	Sugars 4 g	
Monounsaturated Fat 1.0 g	Protein 1 g	

Jícama and Grapefruit Salad with Ancho-Honey Dressing

Serves 4

Ancho peppers are dried poblano peppers. Wrinkled and dark reddish-brown, they add a medium-hot boost to the dressing for this salad, which balances tart vinegar with deeply sweet honey.

DRESSING

- ½ cup water
- 2 ancho peppers, halved lengthwise, seeds and ribs discarded (see Cook's Tip on page 101)
- 2 medium garlic cloves, quartered
- 2 tablespoons white wine vinegar
- 2 tablespoons honey
- 1 tablespoon canola or corn oil
- 1 tablespoon fresh lime juice

SALAD

- 1 pound jícama, peeled and cut into matchstick-size strips
- ½ cup chopped red onion
- ¼ cup chopped fresh cilantro
- 1 large red or pink grapefruit (see Cook's Tip on page 72)

In a small saucepan, bring the water, peppers, and garlic to a boil over high heat. Reduce the heat and simmer for 10 minutes. Transfer the mixture to a food processor or blender (vent the blender lid) and process until smooth.

Add the remaining dressing ingredients. Process until smooth.

In a medium serving bowl, stir together the jícama, onion, and cilantro. Pour the dressing over the mixture, tossing to coat. Cover and refrigerate for 2 to 24 hours.

Just before serving, peel and section the grapefruit. Drain well. Gently stir the grapefruit sections into the salad.

COOK'S TIP ON JÍCAMA: Also called a Mexican potato, jícama is a root vegetable with a thin brown skin and crunchy cream-colored flesh. It has a sweet, nutty flavor and can be eaten raw or cooked. Use jícama as you would carrot and celery sticks, or chop or shred jícama to add to a fresh green salad. Choose bulbs that are firm and free of blemishes. Store whole jícama, unwrapped, in the refrigerator for up to five days. Peel the bulbs just before using them for the freshest flavor. Wrap leftover jícama in plastic wrap and refrigerate for two to three days.

PER SERVING

Calories 170	Cholesterol 0 mg	DIETARY EXCHANGES:
Total Fat 4.5 g	Sodium 11 mg	1 starch
Saturated Fat 0.5 g	Carbohydrates 33 g	1 fruit
Trans Fat 0.0 g	Fiber 9 g	1 vegetable
Polyunsaturated Fat 1.5 g	Sugars 17 g	½ fat
Monounsaturated Fat 2.5 g	Protein 3 g	

Citrus Rice Salad

Serves 6

Orange juice, mandarin oranges, and honey add tang and sweetness to this rice salad that will pair tastefully with Trout Amandine with Orange-Dijon Sauce (page 132).

SALAD

- ¾ cup fresh orange juice
- ¼ cup water
- 1 cup uncooked instant brown rice
- 1 11-ounce can mandarin oranges in juice or water, drained
- ⅓ cup sweetened dried cranberries
- ¼ cup chopped red onion
- ½ medium rib of celery, chopped
- 2 tablespoons finely chopped fresh parsley
- 2 tablespoons chopped fresh basil

DRESSING

- ⅓ cup fresh orange juice
- 1 tablespoon balsamic vinegar
- 2 teaspoons canola or corn oil
- 2 teaspoons honey

In a small saucepan, bring ¾ cup orange juice and the water to a boil over high heat.

Stir in the rice. Reduce the heat and simmer, covered, for 5 minutes. Remove from the heat and stir. Let stand, covered, for 5 minutes.

Meanwhile, in a medium serving bowl, stir together the remaining salad ingredients.

In a small bowl, whisk together the dressing ingredients.

Stir the rice into the salad. Pour the dressing over the salad, tossing gently to coat. Serve at room temperature or cover and refrigerate for up to 24 hours to serve chilled.

COOK'S TIP ON CHOPPING FRESH HERBS: Put herbs in a measuring cup or coffee mug. Use kitchen scissors to snip the herbs until the pieces are the desired fineness.

COOK'S TIP ON MEASURING STICKY FOODS: Lightly spray cups, measuring spoons, and other utensils with cooking spray before filling them with sticky ingredients, such as honey or molasses. The ingredient will slide out and the utensil will be easier to clean.

PER SERVING

Calories 140	Cholesterol 0 mg	DIETARY EXCHANGES:
Total Fat 2.0 g	Sodium 10 mg	1 starch
Saturated Fat 0.0 g	Carbohydrates 28 g	1 fruit
Trans Fat 0.0 g	Fiber 1 g	
Polyunsaturated Fat 0.5 g	Sugars 14 g	
Monounsaturated Fat 1.0 g	Protein 2 g	

Lemon-Curried Black-Eyed Pea Salad

Serves 8

This hearty side salad comes together in the blink of an eye and is a good complement to a simple entrée, such as Crispy Oven-Fried Chicken (page 144) or Spicy Baked Pork Chops (page 208).

DRESSING

2 tablespoons fresh lemon juice
1 tablespoon water
1 teaspoon olive oil (extra virgin preferred)
1 medium garlic clove, minced
½ teaspoon curry powder
½ teaspoon Dijon mustard (lowest sodium available)
⅛ teaspoon pepper

SALAD

1 15.5-ounce can no-salt-added black-eyed peas, rinsed and drained
1 11-ounce can no-salt-added whole-kernel corn, rinsed and drained
½ cup chopped red onion
½ cup thinly sliced celery
1 teaspoon finely shredded lemon zest

In a small bowl, whisk together the dressing ingredients.

In a medium serving bowl, stir together the salad ingredients. Pour the dressing over the salad, tossing gently to coat. Cover and refrigerate for 1 to 24 hours.

COOK'S TIP: Look for canned no-salt-added "fresh" black-eyed peas. They will offer more flavor than dried peas. If you want to use dried black-eyed peas, soak 1 cup peas (sorted for stones and shriveled peas, rinsed, and drained) overnight in enough water to cover. Drain. In a medium saucepan, bring the peas and 3 cups fresh water to a boil over high heat. Reduce the heat and simmer, covered, for 50 minutes to 1 hour, or just until the peas are tender. Drain well in a colander. Proceed as directed.

COOK'S TIP ON ZESTING CITRUS: When zesting citrus with a rasp-style grater, hold the fruit steady and move the grater over the fruit, as if you were filing it. This allows you to see where you are grating, helping you avoid the bitter white pith, and it keeps the zest in the grater rather than scattering it below.

PER SERVING

Calories 90	Cholesterol 0 mg	DIETARY EXCHANGES:
Total Fat 1.0 g	Sodium 13 mg	1 starch
Saturated Fat 0.0 g	Carbohydrates 18 g	
Trans Fat 0.0 g	Fiber 3 g	
Polyunsaturated Fat 0.0 g	Sugars 4 g	
Monounsaturated Fat 0.5 g	Protein 4 g	

Tabbouleh

Serves 6

Make this Middle Eastern dish well in advance—the flavors improve with age. Serve it at room temperature or chilled, by itself, or stuffed into hollowed-out beefsteak tomatoes from your garden.

2 cups fat-free, low-sodium vegetable broth

2 cups water

1 cup uncooked instant, or fine-grain, bulgur

¼ cup fresh lemon juice

1 tablespoon olive oil (extra virgin preferred)

2 medium tomatoes, finely chopped

3 medium green onions, finely chopped

¼ cup finely chopped fresh mint or 1 tablespoon dried mint, crumbled

¼ cup chopped fresh parsley

   Pepper to taste

In a medium saucepan, bring the broth and water to a boil over high heat.

Put the bulgur in a large, nonmetallic, heatproof bowl. Stir in the boiling broth mixture. Let stand, covered, for 1 hour, or until most of the liquid is absorbed. Drain well in a colander. Squeeze out the excess moisture with your hands or by putting the bulgur in cheesecloth or a dish towel, gathering the ends together, and squeezing. Return the bulgur to the large bowl.

In a small bowl, whisk together the lemon juice and oil. Pour over the bulgur.

Gently stir in the remaining ingredients. Cover and refrigerate for at least 1 hour. Serve chilled or bring the salad to room temperature before serving.

....

COOK'S TIP ON BULGUR: Bulgur is a form of whole wheat that's been cleaned, soaked, dried, and cracked into fine, medium, or coarse grains. Nutritious and versatile, bulgur is available at most supermarkets and health food stores.

....

COOK'S TIP ON CITRUS ZEST: Don't let citrus zest go to waste. When using citrus, zest the entire fruit. Separate the zest into ½-teaspoon piles on a plate and place the plate in the freezer. When the zest is frozen, transfer the piles to an airtight container or a resealable plastic freezer bag and return them to the freezer.

COOK'S TIP ON LEMONS: To pick the juiciest lemons, give them a squeeze. Lemons that give under pressure yield more juice than firmer fruit.

PER SERVING

Calories 120	Cholesterol 0 mg	DIETARY EXCHANGES:
Total Fat 2.5 g	Sodium 22 mg	1 starch
Saturated Fat 0.5 g	Carbohydrates 22 g	1 vegetable
Trans Fat 0.0 g	Fiber 6 g	½ fat
Polyunsaturated Fat 0.5 g	Sugars 2 g	
Monounsaturated Fat 1.5 g	Protein 4 g	

Seafood Pasta Salad

Serves 6

If you like pasta salad and tuna salad, then you're sure to love this combination of the two! Each serving provides a whole grain, omega-3 fatty acids, and vegetables. To make it even more wholesome and for a fancier presentation, line a bowl or platter with romaine leaves, spoon the salad over the lettuce, and top with tomato wedges.

10	ounces dried small or medium whole-grain pasta shells
2	4.5-ounce cans very low sodium albacore tuna packed in water, drained and flaked
1	cup frozen green peas, thawed
1	medium red, green, or yellow bell pepper, chopped
1	small red onion, finely chopped
4	or 5 medium radishes, finely chopped
¼	cup chopped fresh basil or 1 tablespoon plus 1 teaspoon dried basil, crumbled
¼	cup chopped fresh parsley
½	cup light Italian salad dressing (lowest sodium available)
½	teaspoon Dijon mustard (lowest sodium available)

Prepare the pasta using the package directions, omitting the salt. Drain well in a colander. Transfer to a large serving bowl.

Stir the tuna, green peas, bell pepper, onion, radishes, basil, and parsley into the pasta.

In a small bowl, whisk together the salad dressing and mustard. Pour over the pasta mixture, stirring gently to coat. Serve at room temperature or cover and refrigerate for 3 to 4 hours.

....

COOK'S TIP: As a change from the tuna listed here, try canned or vacuum-packed salmon or a cooked fish of your choice.

....

PER SERVING

Calories 276	Cholesterol 19 mg	DIETARY EXCHANGES:
Total Fat 5.5 g	Sodium 267 mg	3 starch
Saturated Fat 0.5 g	Carbohydrates 42 g	1½ lean meat
Trans Fat 0.0 g	Fiber 7 g	
Polyunsaturated Fat 2.5 g	Sugars 4 g	
Monounsaturated Fat 1.0 g	Protein 19 g	

Herbed Chicken Salad

Serves 6

This salad is an enticing standalone, but it works equally well as a stuffing for large bell peppers, hollowed-out tomatoes, or even zucchini boats.

SALAD

- 2 cups diced cooked skinless chicken breast, cooked without salt, all visible fat discarded
- ¼ cup fat-free plain yogurt
- ¼ cup light mayonnaise
- 2 medium green onions, thinly sliced
- 1 small carrot, grated
- 2 medium radishes, grated
- 3 tablespoons chopped celery
- 2 tablespoons chopped green bell pepper
- 2 tablespoons chopped fresh parsley
- 1½ tablespoons tarragon vinegar, or 1½ tablespoons plain rice vinegar or white wine vinegar plus ⅛ teaspoon dried tarragon, crumbled
- 1 teaspoon dried Italian seasoning, crumbled
- 1 teaspoon Worcestershire sauce (lowest sodium available)
- ¼ teaspoon pepper, or to taste

....

- 6 large lettuce leaves, such as romaine
- 1 11-ounce can mandarin oranges in juice or water, drained

In a large bowl, stir together the salad ingredients. Cover and refrigerate for at least 1 hour.

Place the lettuce leaves on salad plates. Spoon the salad over the lettuce. Top with the mandarin oranges.

PER SERVING		
Calories 139	Cholesterol 43 mg	DIETARY EXCHANGES:
Total Fat 4.5 g	Sodium 148 mg	½ fruit
Saturated Fat 1.0 g	Carbohydrates 8 g	2 lean meat
Trans Fat 0.0 g	Fiber 2 g	
Polyunsaturated Fat 2.0 g	Sugars 5 g	
Monounsaturated Fat 1.0 g	Protein 16 g	

Roasted Potato and Chicken Salad with Greek Dressing

Serves 6

For a fresh-tasting entrée salad with Mediterranean style, toss warm roasted potatoes with chicken, green beans, roasted bell peppers, and kalamata olives, all blanketed by a lemony garlic dressing.

SALAD

Olive oil cooking spray

1 pound small red potatoes (about 6), unpeeled, cut into ¾-inch cubes

1½ pounds fresh or frozen green beans, trimmed if fresh

2 cups diced cooked skinless chicken breast, cooked without salt, all visible fat discarded

½ cup roasted red bell peppers, drained if bottled, coarsely chopped

¼ cup kalamata olives, coarsely chopped

¼ teaspoon salt

DRESSING

2 tablespoons white wine vinegar

1 teaspoon grated lemon zest

2 tablespoons fresh lemon juice

2 teaspoons light brown sugar

2 teaspoons olive oil (extra virgin preferred)

2 medium garlic cloves, minced

½ teaspoon dried oregano, crumbled

⅛ teaspoon pepper (optional)

Preheat the oven to 400°F. Lightly spray a baking sheet with cooking spray.

Arrange the potatoes in a single layer on the baking sheet. Lightly spray the potatoes with cooking spray. Bake for 35 to 40 minutes, or until the potatoes are golden brown and tender when pierced with the tip of a sharp knife.

Meanwhile, in a large saucepan, bring the green beans and enough water to cover to a boil over high heat. Reduce the heat to medium high and cook for 6 to 8 minutes, or until tender, stirring occasionally. Drain well in a colander. Pat dry with paper towels. Transfer to a large serving bowl.

Gently stir in the potatoes, chicken, roasted peppers, olives, and salt.

In a small bowl, whisk together the dressing ingredients. Pour over the salad, tossing to coat. Serve warm or cover and refrigerate until needed to serve chilled.

PER SERVING

Calories 210
Total Fat 5.5 g
  Saturated Fat 1.0 g
  Trans Fat 0.0 g
  Polyunsaturated Fat 1.0 g
  Monounsaturated Fat 3.0 g

Cholesterol 40 mg
Sodium 278 mg
Carbohydrates 24 g
  Fiber 5 g
  Sugars 6 g
Protein 18 g

DIETARY EXCHANGES:
1 starch
2 vegetable
2 lean meat

Artichoke-Rotini Salad with Chicken

Serves 4

Artichokes are twice as nice in this one-dish meal. They're used as part of the salad dressing and included in the salad so their delightfully sweet aftertaste can really make your mouth sing.

4 ounces dried whole-grain rotini
1 14-ounce can artichoke hearts, drained, with ¼ cup liquid reserved, divided use
¼ cup fresh lemon juice
2 tablespoons dried basil, crumbled
2 medium garlic cloves, minced
¼ teaspoon crushed red pepper flakes
2 cups diced cooked skinless chicken breast, cooked without salt, all visible fat discarded
1 medium red bell pepper, cut into thin strips about 2 inches long
2 tablespoons olive oil (extra virgin preferred)
¼ teaspoon salt
4 large lettuce leaves

Prepare the pasta using the package directions, omitting the salt. Transfer to a colander and rinse with cold water to cool completely. Drain well.

Meanwhile, for the dressing, in a food processor or blender, process half the artichokes, the reserved artichoke liquid, lemon juice, basil, garlic, and red pepper flakes until smooth.

Coarsely chop the remaining artichokes. Transfer to a medium bowl.

Stir the chicken and bell pepper into the chopped artichokes. Stir in the pasta. Pour in the dressing, tossing gently to coat. Gently stir in the oil and salt. Place the lettuce on salad plates. Spoon the salad over the lettuce. Serve immediately.

PER SERVING

Calories 329	Cholesterol 60 mg	DIETARY EXCHANGES:
Total Fat 10.5 g	Sodium 384 mg	1½ starch
Saturated Fat 2.0 g	Carbohydrates 32 g	2 vegetable
Trans Fat 0.0 g	Fiber 6 g	3 lean meat
Polyunsaturated Fat 1.5 g	Sugars 4 g	
Monounsaturated Fat 6.0 g	Protein 29 g	

Greek Chopped Salad

Serves 4

Raid the garden or pay a visit to the farmers' market to get almost all the primary ingredients you'll need for this hearty vegetarian entrée salad.

DRESSING

- 2 tablespoons finely chopped kalamata olives
- 2 tablespoons finely crumbled fat-free feta cheese
- 2 tablespoons olive oil (extra virgin preferred)
- 2 tablespoons fresh lemon juice
- ½ teaspoon dried oregano, crumbled
- ¼ teaspoon pepper

SALAD

- 4 cups coarsely chopped romaine
- 2½ cups no-salt-added chickpeas, rinsed and drained
- 2 cups torn spinach (about 2 ounces)
- 1 small cucumber, quartered lengthwise and sliced crosswise
- 1 large tomato, seeded and chopped
- ½ cup thin strips of red onion
- ½ cup sliced radishes

In a small bowl, whisk together the dressing ingredients.

In a large bowl, toss together the salad ingredients. Pour the dressing over the salad, tossing to coat.

PER SERVING

Calories 273	Cholesterol 0 mg	DIETARY EXCHANGES:
Total Fat 9.5 g	Sodium 195 mg	2 starch
Saturated Fat 1.0 g	Carbohydrates 37 g	1 vegetable
Trans Fat 0.0 g	Fiber 9 g	1 lean meat
Polyunsaturated Fat 1.5 g	Sugars 5 g	1 fat
Monounsaturated Fat 6.5 g	Protein 12 g	

Taco Salad

Serves 4

Add some spice to your life with this southwest-influenced taco salad. The green chiles and jícama strips ramp up the flavor in a healthy way.

- ½ cup fat-free sour cream
- ½ cup salsa (lowest sodium available)
- 2 tablespoons chopped fresh cilantro
- 2 teaspoons salt-free southwest chipotle seasoning blend
- 12 ounces extra-lean ground beef
- ½ cup chopped red onion
- 2 small garlic cloves, minced
- 1 cup canned no-salt-added diced tomatoes, drained
- 1 cup canned no-salt-added pinto beans, rinsed and drained
- ¼ cup chopped canned mild green chiles, drained
- 1 teaspoon chili powder
- ½ teaspoon ground cumin
- ¼ teaspoon pepper
- 2 cups torn romaine
- 1 cup matchstick-size jícama strips
- ¼ cup shredded fat-free Cheddar cheese
- 2 ounces (about 28) baked tortilla chips (lowest sodium available)

In a small bowl, whisk together the sour cream, salsa, cilantro, and seasoning blend. Set aside.

In a large nonstick skillet, cook the beef, onion, and garlic over medium-high heat for 6 minutes, or until the beef is browned on the outside and no longer pink in the center, stirring occasionally to turn and break up the beef.

Reduce the heat to medium. Stir in the tomatoes, beans, chiles, chili powder, cumin, and pepper. Cook for 4 to 5 minutes, or until heated through, stirring occasionally. Remove from the heat.

Stir in ¼ cup of the sour cream mixture. Set aside the remaining mixture.

Place the romaine on plates. Arrange the jícama on the romaine. Spoon the beef mixture over the salads. Sprinkle with the Cheddar. Top with the remaining sour cream mixture. Garnish with the tortilla chips.

PER SERVING

Calories 332	Cholesterol 63 mg	DIETARY EXCHANGES:
Total Fat 5.5 g	Sodium 343 mg	2 starch
Saturated Fat 2.0 g	Carbohydrates 39 g	2 vegetable
Trans Fat 0.0 g	Fiber 7 g	3 lean meat
Polyunsaturated Fat 0.5 g	Sugars 9 g	
Monounsaturated Fat 2.0 g	Protein 29 g	

Macaroni Salad with Ricotta

Serves 4

You'll never think of pasta salad the same way again after you've sampled this recipe. It tastes rich and creamy and has just a little mustardy sass. Serve it with Light and Lemony Spinach Soup (page 52) for a wholesome lunch that won't slow you down.

4 ounces (1½ cups) dried whole-grain macaroni
1 tablespoon fat-free plain yogurt
2 teaspoons yellow mustard (lowest sodium available)
1 cup fat-free ricotta cheese
1 medium green bell pepper, coarsely chopped
2 medium green onions, coarsely chopped
¼ cup sliced or chopped black olives
1 tablespoon chopped fresh parsley
1 teaspoon chopped pimiento, drained
½ teaspoon dried dillweed, crumbled
½ teaspoon dried basil, crumbled
¼ teaspoon pepper (freshly ground preferred)
2 cups mixed salad greens

Prepare the pasta using the package directions, omitting the salt. Transfer to a colander and rinse with cold water to cool completely. Drain well.

In a large bowl, whisk together the yogurt and mustard. Stir in the ricotta until well blended.

Stir in the pasta and the remaining ingredients except the salad greens. Place the greens on salad plates. Top with the pasta mixture.

PER SERVING

Calories 177	Cholesterol 5 mg	DIETARY EXCHANGES:
Total Fat 2.0 g	Sodium 225 mg	1½ starch
Saturated Fat 0.0 g	Carbohydrates 27 g	1 vegetable
Trans Fat 0.0 g	Fiber 5 g	1 lean meat
Polyunsaturated Fat 0.5 g	Sugars 5 g	
Monounsaturated Fat 1.0 g	Protein 13 g	

Creamy Artichoke Dressing

Serves 6

Toss this silky-smooth dressing with spring greens and extra artichokes that you've coarsely chopped. Triple-Pepper and White Bean Soup with Rotini (page 69) is an excellent pairing for a heart-healthy lunch.

½ 14-ounce can artichoke hearts, rinsed and drained, with 1 tablespoon liquid reserved

2 tablespoons fat-free, low-sodium chicken broth

2 tablespoons fresh lemon juice

1 tablespoon olive oil (extra virgin preferred)

2 medium garlic cloves, minced

½ teaspoon Dijon mustard (lowest sodium available)

¼ teaspoon pepper

In a food processor or blender, process all the ingredients, including 1 tablespoon of artichoke liquid, until very smooth. Transfer to a jar with a tight-fitting lid and refrigerate until ready to serve, up to four days.

PER SERVING

Calories 31	Cholesterol 0 mg	DIETARY EXCHANGES:
Total Fat 2.5 g	Sodium 64 mg	½ fat
Saturated Fat 0.5 g	Carbohydrates 2 g	
Trans Fat 0.0 g	Fiber 0 g	
Polyunsaturated Fat 0.0 g	Sugars 0 g	
Monounsaturated Fat 1.5 g	Protein 1 g	

Creamy Herb Dressing

Serves 10

Serve this dressing cold or hot. It can be used as a dip for a host of raw veggies or even low-fat string cheese. Use it to top grilled chicken breasts or baked potatoes.

- ½ cup fat-free plain yogurt
- ½ cup fat-free sour cream
- 1 medium green onion, minced
- 2 tablespoons finely chopped fresh parsley or cilantro
- ½ teaspoon salt-free lemon-herb seasoning blend
- ½ teaspoon honey or sugar
- ¼ teaspoon dried Italian seasoning, crumbled (optional)

In a small bowl, whisk together the yogurt and sour cream.

Whisk in the remaining ingredients.

To serve chilled, cover and refrigerate until ready to use, or up to four days. To serve hot, pour into a small saucepan and cook over medium heat, stirring gently until heated through. Don't allow the dressing to boil.

PER SERVING

Calories 21	Cholesterol 2 mg	DIETARY EXCHANGES:
Total Fat 0.0 g	Sodium 20 mg	Free
Saturated Fat 0.0 g	Carbohydrates 3 g	
Trans Fat 0.0 g	Fiber 0 g	
Polyunsaturated Fat 0.0 g	Sugars 2 g	
Monounsaturated Fat 0.0 g	Protein 2 g	

Gazpacho Dressing

Serves 6

Replacing the cilantro with other herbs, such as parsley, mint, oregano, or tarragon, or with salt-free herb seasoning blend will give you a wide range of flavor choices for this summery salad dressing reminiscent of the popular chilled soup.

6 ounces low-sodium mixed-vegetable juice or low-sodium tomato juice

1 tablespoon very finely chopped onion, any variety

1 tablespoon very finely chopped celery

1 tablespoon very finely chopped bell pepper, any color

1 tablespoon grated carrot

1 tablespoon finely chopped fresh cilantro or 1 teaspoon dried cilantro, crumbled

1 teaspoon fresh lemon juice

½ teaspoon sugar

¼ teaspoon red hot-pepper sauce or ½ teaspoon Worcestershire sauce (lowest sodium available)

Pepper to taste

In a small bowl, whisk together all the ingredients. Cover and refrigerate for at least 2 hours so the flavors blend.

PER SERVING

Calories 9	Cholesterol 0 mg	DIETARY EXCHANGES:
Total Fat 0.0 g	Sodium 20 mg	Free
Saturated Fat 0.0 g	Carbohydrates 2 g	
Trans Fat 0.0 g	Fiber 0 g	
Polyunsaturated Fat 0.0 g	Sugars 2 g	
Monounsaturated Fat 0.0 g	Protein 0 g	

Parmesan-Peppercorn Ranch Dressing

Serves 8

Cool and creamy, this dressing puts the finishing touch on your favorite salad greens. Pack some in a small airtight container along with some raw vegetables for lunchtime dipping.

¾ cup low-fat buttermilk

¼ cup fat-free sour cream

2 tablespoons light mayonnaise

2 tablespoons shredded or grated Parmesan cheese

½ teaspoon dried parsley, crumbled

½ teaspoon dried chives

¼ teaspoon dried oregano, crumbled

¼ teaspoon garlic powder

⅛ teaspoon salt

⅛ teaspoon pepper (coarsely ground preferred)

In a medium bowl, whisk together all the ingredients. Cover and refrigerate for 30 minutes before serving.

PER SERVING

Calories 31	Cholesterol 4 mg	DIETARY EXCHANGES:
Total Fat 1.5 g	Sodium 121 mg	½ fat
Saturated Fat 0.5 g	Carbohydrates 3 g	
Trans Fat 0.0 g	Fiber 0 g	
Polyunsaturated Fat 0.5 g	Sugars 2 g	
Monounsaturated Fat 0.5 g	Protein 2 g	

Tomatillo-Avocado Dressing

Serves 8

You can use this guacamole-like recipe as a salad dressing, condiment, or dip. The flavor of the avocado is enhanced by the broiler-roasted tomatillos, which look like smallish green tomatoes swathed in thin, papery husks.

Cooking spray

6 medium tomatillos, papery husks discarded, each cut in half

1 medium avocado, chopped

1 medium green onion, chopped

2 medium garlic cloves, minced

½ small fresh jalapeño, seeds and ribs discarded, chopped

1 teaspoon sugar

1 teaspoon fresh lemon juice

½ teaspoon ground cumin

½ teaspoon chili powder

¼ teaspoon salt

⅛ teaspoon pepper

Preheat the broiler. Lightly spray the broiler pan with cooking spray. Place the tomatillos with the skin side up on the broiler pan.

Broil 4 to 6 inches from the heat for 5 minutes. Turn over the tomatillos. Broil for 2 to 3 minutes, or until slightly tender. Cover and refrigerate for at least 10 minutes to cool.

In a food processor or blender, process all the ingredients for 1 minute, or until smooth.

....

COOK'S TIP ON HANDLING HOT CHILES: Hot chiles, such as jalapeños, contain oils that can burn your skin, lips, and eyes. Wear disposable gloves or wash your hands thoroughly with warm, soapy water after handling the peppers.

....

PER SERVING

Calories 56	Cholesterol 0 mg	DIETARY EXCHANGES:
Total Fat 4.0 g	Sodium 78 mg	1 vegetable
Saturated Fat 0.5 g	Carbohydrates 5 g	1 fat
Trans Fat 0.0 g	Fiber 3 g	
Polyunsaturated Fat 0.5 g	Sugars 2 g	
Monounsaturated Fat 2.5 g	Protein 1 g	

Citrus-Tarragon Vinaigrette

Serves 8

Pour this light dressing over cooked or raw chilled vegetables. Or use it to accent the juiciness of a sliced heirloom tomato.

⅓ cup canola or corn oil
2 tablespoons fresh lemon juice
2 tablespoons tarragon vinegar
1 teaspoon chopped fresh parsley
½ teaspoon pepper (freshly ground preferred)
¼ teaspoon dry mustard
⅛ teaspoon garlic powder

In a medium bowl, whisk together all the ingredients. Store in a glass container in the refrigerator for up to four days.

PER SERVING		
Calories 86	Cholesterol 0 mg	DIETARY EXCHANGES:
Total Fat 9.5 g	Sodium 0 mg	2 fat
Saturated Fat 0.5 g	Carbohydrates 0 g	
Trans Fat 0.0 g	Fiber 0 g	
Polyunsaturated Fat 2.5 g	Sugars 0 g	
Monounsaturated Fat 6.0 g	Protein 0 g	

Seafood

FISH ROLL-UPS WITH SPINACH 104

FISH FILLETS WITH BROILED-VEGGIE RICE 106

HEARTY FISH CHOWDER 108

CONFETTI CATFISH FILLETS 110

CRUNCHY ITALIAN CATFISH 111

CRISP CATFISH WITH CREOLE SAUCE 112

GRILLED COD WITH ARTICHOKE-HORSERADISH SAUCE 114

BAKED FLOUNDER AND TOMATOES 116

HALIBUT KEBABS 117

POACHED HALIBUT IN ASIAN BROTH 118

CRUNCHY-CRUSTED SALMON 120

BROILED SALMON WITH OLIVE PESTO 122

MEDITERRANEAN GRILLED SALMON 123

SKILLET SALMON WITH BROCCOLI AND RICE 124

SALMON AND ROTINI WITH CHIPOTLE CREAM 125

TILAPIA PICCATA 126

TILAPIA TACOS WITH ROASTED-TOMATO SALSA 128

TILAPIA WITH LEMON-CRUMB TOPPING 130

JAMAICAN JERK TUNA STEAKS 131

TROUT AMANDINE WITH ORANGE-DIJON SAUCE 132

MUSSELS WITH YOGURT-CAPER SAUCE 134

CAJUN RED SCALLOPS 136

SEAFOOD AND LEMON RISOTTO 138

SEARED TUNA WITH MANGO-PEAR SALSA 140

Fish Roll-Ups with Spinach

Serves 6

Pearly white fillets are rolled up with a moist stuffing, coated with a crisp cracker crust, and then broiled to perfection. This mildly flavored entrée pairs well with nearly any side dish, including Red and Green Pilaf (page 264) and Apple-Lemon Carrots (page 255).

    Cooking spray
½ **cup chopped celery**
3 **tablespoons water (plus more as needed)**
2 **tablespoons chopped onion**
3 **slices whole-grain bread (lowest sodium available), lightly toasted and coarsely crumbled**
¼ **cup chopped cooked spinach (4 to 6 ounces fresh)**
½ **teaspoon dried thyme, crumbled**
    Pepper to taste
6 **mild thin fish fillets, such as sole, flounder, or tilapia (about 4 ounces each), rinsed and patted dry**
1 **large egg white, lightly beaten**
¼ **cup fat-free milk**
½ **cup finely crushed whole-grain cracker crumbs (about 14 fat-free, low-sodium whole-grain saltines)**
2 **tablespoons all-purpose flour**
1 **teaspoon chopped fresh parsley**

Preheat the broiler. Soak six wooden toothpicks in cold water for about 10 minutes. Lightly spray the broiler pan and rack with cooking spray.

In a medium saucepan, bring the celery, water, and onion to a boil over medium-high heat. Reduce the heat and simmer, covered, for 3 to 4 minutes, or until the celery is tender and the onion is soft. Remove from the heat.

Stir the bread crumbs, spinach, thyme, and pepper into the celery mixture until combined, adding water if necessary.

Arrange the fish on a work surface. Spoon the stuffing down the middle of each fillet. Starting from a short side, roll up jelly-roll style and secure with a wooden toothpick.

For the coating, in a small shallow bowl, whisk together the egg white and milk. On a plate, stir together the cracker crumbs and flour.

Dip the roll-ups in the egg white mixture and then in the cracker crumb mixture, turning to coat at each step and gently shaking off any excess. Transfer the roll-ups to the broiler rack.

Broil 4 to 5 inches from the heat for 5 to 7 minutes, or until the fish flakes easily when tested with a fork.

Just before serving, remove the toothpicks. Sprinkle the roll-ups with the parsley.

PER SERVING

Calories 152	Cholesterol 44 mg	DIETARY EXCHANGES:
Total Fat 2.5 g	Sodium 415 mg	1 starch
Saturated Fat 0.5 g	Carbohydrates 15 g	3 lean meat
Trans Fat 0.0 g	Fiber 2 g	
Polyunsaturated Fat 0.5 g	Sugars 2 g	
Monounsaturated Fat 0.5 g	Protein 16 g	

Fish Fillets with Broiled-Veggie Rice

Serves 4

The brown rice in this dish picks up a whisper of smokiness from the broiled vegetables. Stovetop Scalloped Tomatoes (page 270) is a pleasing accompaniment and Strawberry Margarita Ice (page 318) brings a cool end to your meal.

1 medium yellow summer squash, cut into ¼-inch rounds
1 medium red bell pepper, cut into ¼-inch strips
1 medium onion, cut into ¼-inch strips
2 teaspoons olive oil, 2 teaspoons olive oil, and 2 teaspoons olive oil (extra virgin preferred), divided use
½ cup uncooked quick-cooking brown rice
2 tablespoons chopped fresh basil or chopped fresh parsley
1 teaspoon grated lemon zest
2 tablespoons fresh lemon juice
  Cooking spray
4 mild thin fish fillets, such as sole, flounder, or tilapia (about 4 ounces each), rinsed and patted dry
1 teaspoon reduced-sodium seafood seasoning blend
⅛ teaspoon salt

Preheat the broiler. Line a broiler-safe baking sheet with aluminum foil.

Put the squash, bell pepper, and onion on the baking sheet. Pour 2 teaspoons oil over the vegetables. Toss gently to coat. Arrange the vegetables in a single layer.

Broil at least 4 inches from the heat for 9 to 10 minutes, or until richly browned on the edges. Keeping the cooked vegetables on the aluminum foil, remove them from the baking sheet and pour onto a cutting board. Coarsely chop.

Meanwhile, prepare the rice using the package directions, omitting the salt and margarine.

Stir the broiled vegetables, basil, and lemon zest into the cooked rice. Cover to keep warm.

Line the baking sheet with another sheet of aluminum foil. Lightly spray the foil with cooking spray.

Arrange the fish in a single layer on the baking sheet. Spoon 2 teaspoons oil over the fish. Sprinkle the seasoning blend and salt over the fish.

Broil about 4 inches from the heat for 5 minutes, or until the fish flakes easily when tested with a fork.

Serve the fish with the rice mixture. Just before serving, spoon the lemon juice and drizzle the remaining 2 teaspoons oil over the fish.

PER SERVING

Calories 207
Total Fat 9.5 g
  Saturated Fat 1.5 g
  Trans Fat 0.0 g
  Polyunsaturated Fat 1.0 g
  Monounsaturated Fat 5.5 g

Cholesterol 51 mg
Sodium 508 mg
Carbohydrates 15 g
  Fiber 3 g
  Sugars 5 g
Protein 16 g

DIETARY EXCHANGES:
½ starch
1 vegetable
3 lean meat

Hearty Fish Chowder

Serves 6

You can almost feel the salt in the air off the bay in every spoonful of this satisfying entrée soup. Serve it with Speckled Spoon Bread (page 280) for a New England–style meal.

3 tablespoons light tub margarine

2 medium onions, diced

1 cup sliced button mushrooms

1 cup chopped green bell pepper

½ cup all-purpose flour

4 cups fat-free milk

1 pound firm white fish fillets, such as halibut, rinsed, patted dry, and coarsely chopped

¼ cup chopped fresh parsley

1 tablespoon tamari sauce (lowest sodium available)

Pepper to taste (freshly ground preferred)

2 medium Yukon gold potatoes, peeled and cubed, cooked until tender

½ cup dry sherry or 100% apple cider

In a medium skillet, melt the margarine over medium-high heat, swirling to coat the bottom. Cook the onions, mushrooms, and bell pepper for 4 minutes, or until the onions are soft, stirring frequently.

Add the flour, stirring until well blended. Gradually pour in the milk, stirring constantly until the mixture is smooth.

Increase the heat to high. Stir in the fish, parsley, tamari sauce, and pepper. Bring to a boil. Reduce the heat and simmer for 10 minutes, or until the fish flakes easily when tested with a fork.

Stir in the potatoes and sherry. Cook for 3 minutes, or until the chowder is heated through.

cook's tip on tamari sauce: Tamari is a style of soy sauce that is thicker and darker, with a rich, mellow flavor. It's often wheat-free, so it's perfect for people avoiding gluten. Look for it in the Asian food aisle of the supermarket, near the soy sauce.

cook's tip on sherry: When a recipe calls for sherry, be sure to use dry sherry and not cooking sherry, which contains added sodium.

PER SERVING

Calories 266	Cholesterol 40 mg	DIETARY EXCHANGES:
Total Fat 3.5 g	Sodium 276 mg	1 starch
Saturated Fat 0.5 g	Carbohydrates 32 g	½ fat-free milk
Trans Fat 0.0 g	Fiber 3 g	1 vegetable
Polyunsaturated Fat 1.0 g	Sugars 13 g	2 lean meat
Monounsaturated Fat 1.5 g	Protein 23 g	

Confetti Catfish Fillets

Serves 6

Bright red bell pepper and vivid green chives and parsley add flashes of color to this entrée. The flavor combination works well with any firm white fish. This is truly a dish worth celebrating!

Cooking spray
1½ teaspoons canola or corn oil
½ cup finely chopped onion
¼ cup diced red bell pepper
2 tablespoons chopped fresh chives or minced green onion (green part only)
1 tablespoon chopped fresh parsley
1½ slices whole-grain bread (lowest sodium available)
1 teaspoon grated lemon zest
1 tablespoon fresh lemon juice
6 firm white fish fillets, such as catfish or mahi mahi (about 4 ounces each), rinsed and patted dry
¼ teaspoon salt
Pepper to taste (white preferred)

Preheat the oven to 400°F. Lightly spray a 13 x 9 x 2-inch baking dish with cooking spray.

In a small nonstick skillet, heat the oil over medium-high heat, swirling to coat the bottom. Cook the onion and bell pepper for 3 minutes, or until the onion is soft, stirring frequently. Stir in the chives and parsley. Cook for 2 minutes. Remove from the heat.

In a food processor or blender, process the bread into fine crumbs. Stir the crumbs and lemon zest into the onion mixture until combined.

Arrange the fish in the baking dish. Sprinkle the lemon juice, salt, and pepper over the fish. Spread the crumb mixture over the top.

Bake the fish for 10 minutes per inch of thickness at the thickest point, or until it flakes easily when tested with a fork.

PER SERVING

Calories 144	Cholesterol 66 mg	DIETARY EXCHANGES:
Total Fat 4.5 g	Sodium 172 mg	½ starch
Saturated Fat 1.0 g	Carbohydrates 5 g	3 lean meat
Trans Fat 0.0 g	Fiber 1 g	
Polyunsaturated Fat 1.5 g	Sugars 1 g	
Monounsaturated Fat 1.5 g	Protein 20 g	

Crunchy Italian Catfish

Serves 4

You can easily eliminate unwanted added sodium by making your own fresh bread crumbs. Try this entrée with Roasted Brussels Sprouts (page 252), which cooks at the same temperature. Just pop the brussels sprouts in the oven while you're prepping the fish to have everything done at the same time.

Cooking spray
4 catfish or other mild, thin fish fillets (about 4 ounces each), rinsed and patted dry
½ medium lemon, 1 teaspoon grated lemon zest, and 1 medium lemon, cut into 4 wedges, divided use
3 slices reduced-calorie whole-grain bread (lowest sodium available), coarsely torn
2 tablespoons chopped fresh parsley
1 tablespoon shredded or grated Parmesan cheese
1 teaspoon dried oregano, crumbled
⅛ teaspoon cayenne
⅛ teaspoon salt
2 tablespoons olive oil

Preheat the oven to 400°F. Line a baking sheet with aluminum foil. Lightly spray the foil with cooking spray.

Place the fish on the baking sheet. Squeeze the half lemon over the fish.

In a food processor or blender, process the bread, pulsing to make coarse crumbs. Transfer to a medium bowl.

Stir in the parsley, Parmesan, lemon zest, oregano, cayenne, and salt.

Stir in the oil. Sprinkle the crumb mixture over the fish. Bake for 12 to 15 minutes, or until the fish flakes easily when tested with a fork. Serve with the remaining lemon wedges.

PER SERVING

Calories 206	Cholesterol 67 mg	DIETARY EXCHANGES:
Total Fat 11.0 g	Sodium 230 mg	½ starch
Saturated Fat 2.0 g	Carbohydrates 8 g	3 lean meat
Trans Fat 0.0 g	Fiber 3 g	
Polyunsaturated Fat 1.5 g	Sugars 1 g	
Monounsaturated Fat 6.0 g	Protein 21 g	

Crisp Catfish with Creole Sauce

Serves 4

This catfish boasts a quick marinade of spicy buttermilk, a crisp golden coating, and a horseradish-spiked sauce. Serve with Sautéed Greens and Cabbage (page 261) and Twice-Baked Potatoes and Herbs (page 262). While the fish is marinating, put the potatoes in the oven. They cook at the same temperature as the fish, so their cooking times can easily overlap.

¼ cup low-fat buttermilk

⅛ teaspoon cayenne

4 catfish fillets (about 4 ounces each), rinsed and patted dry

SAUCE

⅓ cup no-salt-added tomato sauce

1 medium rib of celery, finely chopped

1 medium green onion, thinly sliced

1 teaspoon bottled white horseradish, drained

1 teaspoon fresh lemon juice

¼ teaspoon salt

. . . .

Cooking spray

1½ cups cornflake cereal, crushed

⅓ cup yellow cornmeal

In a large shallow dish, stir together the buttermilk and cayenne. Add the fish, turning to coat. Cover and refrigerate for 15 minutes to 1 hour, turning occasionally.

Meanwhile, in a small bowl, stir together the sauce ingredients. Cover and refrigerate until needed, up to four days.

Preheat the oven to 425°F. Lightly spray a baking sheet with cooking spray.

In a medium shallow bowl, stir together the crushed cereal and the cornmeal.

Set the dish with the fish, the bowl with the cereal mixture, and the baking sheet in a row, assembly-line fashion. Drain the fish, discarding the marinade. Dip the fish in the cornflake mixture, turning to coat and gently shaking off any excess. Place on the baking sheet. Lightly spray the top of the fish with cooking spray.

Bake for 10 to 12 minutes, or until the fish flakes easily when tested with a fork.

Meanwhile, remove the sauce from the refrigerator if you want to serve it at room temperature rather than chilled. Spoon the sauce over the fish.

PER SERVING

Calories 197	Cholesterol 66 mg	DIETARY EXCHANGES:
Total Fat 3.5 g	Sodium 288 mg	1½ starch
Saturated Fat 1.0 g	Carbohydrates 21 g	3 lean meat
Trans Fat 0.0 g	Fiber 2 g	
Polyunsaturated Fat 1.0 g	Sugars 3 g	
Monounsaturated Fat 1.0 g	Protein 21 g	

Grilled Cod with Artichoke-Horseradish Sauce

Serves 4

Mild-tasting cod is elevated when it's joined by a creamy yet chunky sauce with a distinct flavor. Serve the fish over a bed of quinoa or another whole grain along with grilled asparagus for a complete meal.

1	tablespoon light tub margarine
½	cup chopped shallots or onion
2	medium garlic cloves, minced
2	tablespoons all-purpose flour
⅛	teaspoon salt
⅛	teaspoon pepper
1	12-ounce can fat-free evaporated milk
9	ounces frozen artichoke hearts, thawed, drained, and halved
1	to 2 tablespoons grated fresh or bottled white horseradish, drained
1	tablespoon chopped fresh oregano or 1 teaspoon dried oregano, crumbled
	Cooking spray
4	cod or halibut fillets (about 4 ounces each), rinsed and patted dry

In a medium saucepan, melt the margarine over medium heat, swirling to coat the bottom. Cook the shallots and garlic for 5 minutes, or until the shallots are soft, stirring occasionally.

Stir in the flour, salt, and pepper.

Pour in the milk all at once, whisking constantly. Cook for 5 to 10 minutes, or until the sauce is thickened and bubbly, whisking constantly. Continue cooking for 1 minute, whisking constantly.

Stir in the artichokes, horseradish, and oregano. Cook for 3 to 5 minutes, or until heated through, stirring constantly. Remove from the heat. Cover to keep warm.

Lightly spray the grill rack or broiler pan and rack with cooking spray. Preheat the grill on medium high or preheat the broiler.

Grill the fish, or broil it about 4 inches from the heat, for 7 minutes. Turn over the fish. Grill or broil for 5 to 7 minutes, or until the fish flakes easily when tested with a fork.

Just before serving, spoon the sauce over the fish.

PER SERVING

Calories 235	Cholesterol 52 mg	DIETARY EXCHANGES:
Total Fat 2.0 g	Sodium 292 mg	1 fat-free milk
Saturated Fat 0.5 g	Carbohydrates 24 g	2 vegetable
Trans Fat 0.0 g	Fiber 5 g	3 lean meat
Polyunsaturated Fat 0.5 g	Sugars 12 g	
Monounsaturated Fat 1.0 g	Protein 29 g	

Baked Flounder and Tomatoes

Serves 6

Nestled under a golden bread-crumb topping are slices of juicy tomato and lemon-marinated fish baked to perfection in just minutes. As a complementary side dish, prepare Stuffed Zucchini (page 271), which bakes at the same temperature. Just put the side dish in the oven half an hour before the fish and they'll be ready at the same time.

Cooking spray
1½ cups water
2 tablespoons fresh lemon juice
6 flounder or cod fillets (about 4 ounces each), rinsed
Pepper to taste (freshly ground preferred)
2 large tomatoes, sliced
½ medium green bell pepper, minced
2 tablespoons minced onion
½ cup whole-wheat panko (Japanese-style bread crumbs)
1 tablespoon canola or corn oil
½ teaspoon dried basil, crumbled

Preheat the oven to 350°F. Lightly spray a 13 x 9 x 2-inch baking dish with cooking spray.

In a large shallow dish, whisk together the water and lemon juice. Add the fish, turning to coat. Cover and refrigerate for 10 minutes.

Drain the fish, discarding the marinade. Transfer the fish to the baking dish. Sprinkle the pepper over the fish. Arrange the tomato slices on the fish. Sprinkle the bell pepper and onion over the tomatoes.

In a small bowl, stir together the panko, oil, and basil. Spread over the fish and vegetables. Bake for 10 to 15 minutes, or until the fish flakes easily when tested with a fork.

PER SERVING

Calories 163	Cholesterol 54 mg	DIETARY EXCHANGES:
Total Fat 4.0 g	Sodium 105 mg	½ starch
Saturated Fat 0.5 g	Carbohydrates 8 g	3 lean meat
Trans Fat 0.0 g	Fiber 2 g	
Polyunsaturated Fat 1.0 g	Sugars 2 g	
Monounsaturated Fat 2.0 g	Protein 23 g	

Halibut Kebabs

Serves 4

Halibut easily soaks up this quick-to-prepare marinade, providing a depth of Mediterranean flavor. While the fish is marinating, prepare a side dish or two, such as Fennel-Orange Salad (page 74) or Citrus Rice Salad (page 82), because once the fish is under the broiler, it will be done in no time.

MARINADE

¼ cup fresh lemon juice

¼ cup olive oil

3 medium shallots, thinly sliced

1 teaspoon dried Italian seasoning, crumbled

½ teaspoon dried thyme, crumbled

. . . .

1 pound halibut fillets, rinsed and patted dry, cut into 16 1-inch cubes

Cooking spray

½ large red onion, cut into 20 1-inch squares

1 medium lemon, cut into 4 wedges

In a large shallow dish, stir together the marinade ingredients. Add the fish to the marinade, turning to coat. Cover and refrigerate for 15 minutes to 1 hour, turning occasionally.

Meanwhile, soak four 12-inch wooden skewers in cold water for at least 10 minutes to keep them from charring, or use metal skewers.

Preheat the broiler. Lightly spray the broiler pan and rack with cooking spray.

Drain the fish, discarding the marinade. Thread each skewer with 5 onion squares and 4 fish cubes, alternating the ingredients.

Broil the kebabs about 4 inches from the heat for 2 to 2½ minutes on each side, or until the fish flakes easily when tested with a fork.

Serve the kebabs with the lemon wedges.

PER SERVING

Calories 111	Cholesterol 56 mg	DIETARY EXCHANGES:
Total Fat 1.5 g	Sodium 78 mg	3 lean meat
Saturated Fat 0.5 g	Carbohydrates 2 g	
Trans Fat 0.0 g	Fiber 0 g	
Polyunsaturated Fat 0.5 g	Sugars 1 g	
Monounsaturated Fat 0.5 g	Protein 21 g	

Poached Halibut in Asian Broth

Serves 4

Asian broths are known for their well-seasoned depth of flavor. Thanks especially to the ginger and heat of cayenne, this one is no exception, giving this fish dish a delectable taste and aroma. The brilliant orange carrot confetti is a festive finishing touch that adds to the mouthfeel of the dish.

BROTH

- 3 cups fat-free, low-sodium chicken broth
- 2 tablespoons dry sherry (optional)
- 2 tablespoons soy sauce (lowest sodium available)
- 2 lemon slices
- 3 thin slices peeled gingerroot
- ⅛ teaspoon cayenne

. . . .

- 4 halibut or other mild, thick fish fillets (about 4 ounces each), rinsed
- 5 or 6 medium green onions (green part only), cut into 1-inch pieces
- 1 medium red bell pepper, cut into 1 x ¼-inch strips
- 1 medium rib of celery, cut into 1 x ¼-inch strips
- ½ teaspoon toasted sesame oil
- 1 medium carrot, grated
- Pepper to taste

In a wok or large skillet, stir together the broth ingredients. Cook, covered, over medium heat until just boiling.

Gently place the fish in the broth. If necessary, pour in enough water to barely cover the fish. Reduce the heat and simmer for about 10 minutes per inch of thickness at the thickest point, or just until the fish flakes easily when tested with a fork. Using a slotted spatula, transfer the fish to soup bowls.

Return the liquid to a boil. Stir in the green onions, bell pepper, and celery.

Cook for 2 to 3 minutes, or until the bell pepper and celery are tender-crisp, stirring occasionally. Discard the lemon and gingerroot.

Using a slotted spoon, transfer the vegetables to the soup bowls. Stir the sesame oil into the broth. Pour into the bowls. Sprinkle each serving with the carrot and pepper.

PER SERVING

Calories 158	Cholesterol 56 mg	DIETARY EXCHANGES:
Total Fat 2.5 g	Sodium 346 mg	1 vegetable
Saturated Fat 0.5 g	Carbohydrates 8 g	3 lean meat
Trans Fat 0.0 g	Fiber 3 g	
Polyunsaturated Fat 0.5 g	Sugars 5 g	
Monounsaturated Fat 1.0 g	Protein 24 g	

Crunchy-Crusted Salmon

Serves 4

Buttermilk helps tenderize the salmon and keep it moist as it bakes. The coating of whole-grain oatmeal and almonds adds a nutty crunch. Wilted Spinach (page 268) is a quick complement for this fast-cooking entrée and provides a nutritious and colorful bed on which the fish can be served.

⅓ cup low-fat buttermilk
4 salmon fillets (about 4 ounces each), rinsed

COATING

½ cup uncooked quick-cooking oatmeal
¼ cup sliced almonds
1 teaspoon dried oregano, crumbled
½ teaspoon garlic powder
½ teaspoon paprika
¼ teaspoon salt
¼ teaspoon pepper
. . . .
Cooking spray

Pour the buttermilk into a large shallow dish. Add the fish, turning to coat. Cover and refrigerate for 10 minutes to 1 hour, turning occasionally.

Meanwhile, in a medium shallow dish, stir together the coating ingredients. Set aside.

Preheat the oven to 400°F. Lightly spray a baking sheet with cooking spray.

Set the large shallow dish, the medium shallow dish, and the baking sheet in a row, assembly-line fashion. Drain the fish, discarding the buttermilk. Dip the fish in the oatmeal mixture, turning to coat and gently shaking off any excess. Place on the baking sheet.

Bake for 10 to 12 minutes, or until the fish is the desired doneness.

COOK'S TIP: For variety, substitute tilapia or catfish fillets for the salmon.

COOK'S TIP ON BUTTERMILK: If you don't have any buttermilk for this or any other recipe, you can easily make your own substitute. Stir together ⅓ cup fat-free milk and 1 teaspoon lemon juice or vinegar. Let it stand for 10 minutes.

PER SERVING

Calories 228	Cholesterol 53 mg	DIETARY EXCHANGES:
Total Fat 8.5 g	Sodium 253 mg	½ starch
Saturated Fat 1.5 g	Carbohydrates 10 g	3 lean meat
Trans Fat 0.0 g	Fiber 2 g	
Polyunsaturated Fat 2.0 g	Sugars 1 g	
Monounsaturated Fat 3.5 g	Protein 27 g	

Broiled Salmon with Olive Pesto

Serves 4

An aromatic pesto accented with black olives and citrus makes the flavor profile of this dish more sophisticated than your average broiled salmon. Not only is it packed with salmon's heart-healthy omega 3s, it's also super fast to cook.

Cooking spray
1 cup loosely packed fresh basil
2 tablespoons pine nuts
2 tablespoons sliced black olives
1 teaspoon grated orange zest
2 tablespoons fresh orange juice
1 tablespoon light mayonnaise
2 teaspoons olive oil
2 medium garlic cloves, minced
4 salmon fillets (about 4 ounces each), rinsed and patted dry

Preheat the broiler. Lightly spray the broiler pan with cooking spray.

In a food processor or blender, process the remaining ingredients except the fish for 15 to 20 seconds, or until slightly chunky.

Place the fish on the broiler pan. Using a pastry brush or spoon, spread the basil mixture over both sides of the fish.

Broil the fish about 4 inches from the heat for 5 to 6 minutes. Turn over the fish. Broil for 4 to 5 minutes, or until the desired doneness.

PER SERVING

Calories 205	Cholesterol 53 mg	DIETARY EXCHANGES:
Total Fat 10.5 g	Sodium 149 mg	3 lean meat
Saturated Fat 1.5 g	Carbohydrates 3 g	
Trans Fat 0.0 g	Fiber 1 g	
Polyunsaturated Fat 2.5 g	Sugars 1 g	
Monounsaturated Fat 4.5 g	Protein 25 g	

Mediterranean Grilled Salmon

Serves 6

You'll need a bit of time for marinating, but the results will be well worth it. The heady aroma of fresh herbs and the zing of lemon turn this salmon into a simple but succulent dish. Serve with quinoa or farro and grilled asparagus.

MARINADE

- 1 medium Italian plum (Roma) tomato, finely chopped
- 2 tablespoons red wine vinegar
- 1 tablespoon chopped fresh rosemary or 1 teaspoon dried rosemary, crushed
- 1 tablespoon chopped fresh sage or 1 teaspoon dried rubbed sage
- 2 teaspoons olive oil
- 1 teaspoon grated lemon zest
- ¼ teaspoon pepper

....

- 6 salmon fillets (about 4 ounces each), rinsed
  Cooking spray

In a large shallow dish, stir together the marinade ingredients. Add the fish, turning to coat. Cover and refrigerate for 30 minutes to 2 hours, turning occasionally.

Meanwhile, lightly spray the grill rack or broiler pan and rack with cooking spray. Preheat the grill on medium high or preheat the broiler.

Drain the fish, discarding the marinade. Grill the fish, or broil it about 4 inches from the heat, for 5 to 6 minutes. Turn over the fish. Grill or broil for 4 to 5 minutes, or until the fish is the desired doneness.

PER SERVING

Calories 144	Cholesterol 52 mg	DIETARY EXCHANGES:
Total Fat 5.0 g	Sodium 85 mg	3 lean meat
Saturated Fat 1.0 g	Carbohydrates 0 g	
Trans Fat 0.0 g	Fiber 0 g	
Polyunsaturated Fat 1.0 g	Sugars 0 g	
Monounsaturated Fat 1.5 g	Protein 23 g	

Skillet Salmon with Broccoli and Rice

Serves 4

This dish is ideal for a busy night because it combines quick-cooking brown rice and salmon in a pouch, which needs no cooking at all.

1	teaspoon olive oil
2	medium garlic cloves, minced
12	ounces broccoli florets
1½	cups fat-free, low-sodium chicken broth
1	teaspoon grated lemon zest
¼	teaspoon pepper
1	cup uncooked quick-cooking brown rice
2	5-ounce vacuum-sealed pouches boneless, skinless pink salmon, flaked
1	cup cherry tomatoes, halved
¼	cup fresh basil, coarsely chopped

In a large deep skillet, heat the oil over medium heat, swirling to coat the bottom. Cook the garlic for 10 to 15 seconds. Watch carefully so it doesn't burn.

Stir in the broccoli. Increase the heat to medium high and cook for 2 to 3 minutes, or until tender-crisp, stirring occasionally.

Stir in the broth, lemon zest, and pepper. Bring to a simmer, stirring occasionally.

Stir in the rice. Reduce the heat and simmer, covered, for 5 minutes. Remove from the heat.

Let stand, covered, for 5 minutes, or until the rice is tender and all the liquid is absorbed.

Stir in the salmon, tomatoes, and basil.

PER SERVING

Calories 219	Cholesterol 25 mg	DIETARY EXCHANGES:
Total Fat 5.0 g	Sodium 416 mg	1 starch
Saturated Fat 1.5 g	Carbohydrates 26 g	2 vegetable
Trans Fat 0.0 g	Fiber 4 g	2 lean meat
Polyunsaturated Fat 1.0 g	Sugars 3 g	
Monounsaturated Fat 1.5 g	Protein 19 g	

Salmon and Rotini with Chipotle Cream

Serves 4

The chipotle pepper gives this seafood entrée a smoky blast of heat. Serve it with mixed salad greens tossed with Gazpacho Dressing (page 99).

6 ounces dried whole-grain rotini
12 ounces green beans, trimmed and halved
½ cup fat-free sour cream
¼ cup light mayonnaise
½ to 1 chipotle pepper canned in adobo sauce, minced (see Cook's Tip on page 101), and 2 teaspoons adobo sauce, divided use
¼ teaspoon garlic powder
¼ teaspoon ground cumin
1 5-ounce vacuum-sealed pouch boneless, skinless pink salmon, flaked
2 to 3 tablespoons chopped fresh cilantro

Prepare the pasta using the package directions, omitting the salt. About 3 minutes before the end of the cooking time, stir in the green beans. Drain the pasta and green beans well in a colander.

Meanwhile, in a large shallow bowl, whisk together the sour cream, mayonnaise, chipotle pepper, adobo sauce, garlic powder, and cumin.

Gently stir in the pasta mixture.

Sprinkle with the salmon and cilantro. Don't stir.

PER SERVING

Calories 287	Cholesterol 23 mg	DIETARY EXCHANGES:
Total Fat 6.0 g	Sodium 441 mg	2½ starch
Saturated Fat 1.0 g	Carbohydrates 45 g	1 vegetable
Trans Fat 0.0 g	Fiber 7 g	1 lean meat
Polyunsaturated Fat 3.0 g	Sugars 7 g	
Monounsaturated Fat 1.0 g	Protein 16 g	

Tilapia Piccata

Lemon and capers enhance the mild taste of tilapia with their tart and briny flavors. Try this dish over whole-grain pasta or a bed of lightly steamed spinach. *Buon appetito!*

1   tablespoon all-purpose flour and ⅓ cup all-purpose flour, divided use

1   packet (1 teaspoon) salt-free instant chicken bouillon

¾   cup water

¼   cup dry white wine (regular or nonalcoholic)

1   tablespoon fresh lemon juice

1   tablespoon capers, drained

⅛   teaspoon salt

⅛   teaspoon pepper

4   tilapia or other mild, thin fish fillets (about 4 ounces each), rinsed and patted dry

1   tablespoon olive oil
    Cooking spray

2   teaspoons light tub margarine

1   medium lemon, cut into 4 wedges

In a small bowl, whisk together 1 tablespoon flour and the bouillon. Gradually pour in the water, whisking until smooth. Whisk in the wine and lemon juice. Stir in the capers. Set aside.

In a shallow dish, stir together the remaining ⅓ cup flour, salt, and pepper. Dip the fish in the flour mixture, turning to coat and shaking off any excess. Transfer to a large plate.

In a large nonstick skillet, heat the oil over medium-high heat, swirling to coat the bottom. Cook the fish for 3 minutes. Remove from the heat.

Lightly spray the top of the fish with cooking spray. Turn over the fish. Cook for 2 to 3 minutes, or until the fish flakes easily when tested with a fork. Transfer the fish to a separate large plate.

Pour the bouillon mixture into the skillet. Bring to a boil, still over medium-high heat, whisking constantly. Reduce the heat and simmer for 3 to 5 minutes, or until slightly thickened, whisking frequently.

With the heat on low, whisk in the margarine until melted. Return the fish to the skillet. Spoon the sauce over the fish. Simmer for 1 to 2 minutes, or until the fish and sauce are heated through.

Transfer the fish to plates. Spoon the sauce over the fish. Serve with the lemon wedges.

PER SERVING

Calories 205	Cholesterol 57 mg	DIETARY EXCHANGES:
Total Fat 6.0 g	Sodium 213 mg	½ starch
Saturated Fat 1.0 g	Carbohydrates 11 g	3 lean meat
Trans Fat 0.0 g	Fiber 0 g	
Polyunsaturated Fat 1.0 g	Sugars 0 g	
Monounsaturated Fat 3.5 g	Protein 24 g	

Tilapia Tacos with Roasted-Tomato Salsa

Serves 4

A dusting of cornmeal gives these lime-marinated tilapia fillets a lightly crunchy crust when browned. Homemade salsa adds a touch of smoky heat. *(See photo on cover.)*

- 4 tilapia or other mild, thin fish fillets (about 4 ounces each), rinsed and patted dry
- 2 tablespoons fresh lime juice
- 1 teaspoon chili powder
- 1 teaspoon garlic powder
- 1 teaspoon onion powder
- ¼ teaspoon salt
  Cooking spray
- 1 small fresh jalapeño, seeds and ribs discarded, halved lengthwise (see Cook's Tip on page 101)
- 2 medium green onions
- 1 14.5-ounce can no-salt-added fire-roasted diced tomatoes, drained
- 2 to 3 tablespoons coarsely chopped fresh cilantro
- ¼ cup plus 2 tablespoons yellow cornmeal
- 2 teaspoons olive oil
- 8 6-inch corn tortillas
- 2 cups shredded cabbage
- 2 to 3 medium radishes, thinly sliced (optional)
- 1 medium lime, cut into 4 wedges

Put the fish in a large shallow casserole dish. Sprinkle the lime juice over both sides of the fish.

In a small bowl, stir together the chili powder, garlic powder, onion powder, and salt. Sprinkle over both sides of the fish. Cover and refrigerate for 15 minutes to 1 hour. Using your fingertips, gently press the mixture so it adheres to the fish.

Meanwhile, lightly spray the broiler pan with cooking spray. Preheat the broiler.

Put the jalapeño on the broiler pan with the cut side down. Broil for 3 minutes. Using tongs, turn over the jalapeño. Put the green onions on the pan. Broil for 3 minutes, or until the jalapeño and green onions are charred.

In a food processor or blender, process the tomatoes, green onions, jalapeño, and cilantro for 10 to 15 seconds, or until the desired consistency. Transfer to a small bowl. Cover and refrigerate until serving time.

Put the cornmeal in a medium shallow bowl.

Drain the fish, discarding the marinade. Dip the fish in the cornmeal, turning to coat and gently shaking off any excess. Using your fingertips, gently press the coating so it adheres to the fish. Transfer the fish to a plate.

In a large nonstick skillet, heat the oil over medium-high heat, swirling to coat the bottom. Cook the fish for 4 to 5 minutes on each side, or until it flakes easily when tested with a fork. Transfer to a cutting board. Cut each fillet in half.

Warm the tortillas using the package directions.

Place one piece of fish in the center of each tortilla. Spoon the salsa over the fish. Sprinkle with the cabbage and radishes. Fold each tortilla in half. Serve with the lime wedges.

PER SERVING

Calories 284	Cholesterol 57 mg	DIETARY EXCHANGES:
Total Fat 5.5 g	Sodium 283 mg	1½ starch
Saturated Fat 1.0 g	Carbohydrates 34 g	2 vegetable
Trans Fat 0.0 g	Fiber 5 g	3 lean meat
Polyunsaturated Fat 1.0 g	Sugars 6 g	
Monounsaturated Fat 2.5 g	Protein 27 g	

Tilapia with Lemon-Crumb Topping

Serves 4

Fish in a flash! Here's a dish that looks and tastes so much fresher than frozen, breaded fish fillets. And it's in and out of your microwave and table-ready in just seven minutes.

¼	teaspoon salt
4	tilapia or other mild white fish fillets (about 4 ounces each), rinsed and patted dry
8	large fat-free, low-sodium whole-grain crackers
2	tablespoons light tub margarine
1	tablespoon chopped fresh parsley
1½	teaspoons fresh lemon juice

Sprinkle the salt over both sides of the fish. Transfer the fish to a microwaveable baking dish with a lid. Set aside.

In a food processor or blender, process the crackers into fine crumbs.

In a small microwaveable bowl, microwave the margarine on 50 percent power (medium) for 30 seconds, or until melted. Remove from the microwave. Stir the margarine. Add the cracker crumbs, parsley, and lemon juice, stirring until the mixture is well combined. Sprinkle over the fish.

Microwave the fish, covered, on 100 percent power (high) for 6 to 7 minutes, or until it flakes easily when tested with a fork. Remove from the microwave. Carefully uncover the dish away from you (to prevent steam burns).

PER SERVING

Calories 165	Cholesterol 57 mg	DIETARY EXCHANGES:
Total Fat 5.5 g	Sodium 265 mg	½ starch
Saturated Fat 1.0 g	Carbohydrates 6 g	3 lean meat
Trans Fat 0.0 g	Fiber 1 g	
Polyunsaturated Fat 1.5 g	Sugars 0 g	
Monounsaturated Fat 2.5 g	Protein 24 g	

Jamaican Jerk Tuna Steaks

Serves 4

For a meal that will make you feel as if you're on an island vacation, serve this grilled or broiled jerk-seasoned fish over brown rice flavored with pineapple. To finish off your tropical dinner, try Bananas Foster Plus (page 315).

    8 ounces pineapple chunks canned in their own juice, drained and juice reserved

    2 ounces diced pimiento, drained

    2 medium green onions, thinly sliced

    ¾ cup uncooked quick-cooking brown rice

      Cooking spray

    1 tablespoon olive oil

    4 tuna steaks (about 4 ounces each), about 1 inch thick, rinsed and patted dry

    ¼ teaspoon dried thyme, crumbled

    ¼ teaspoon ground allspice

    ¼ teaspoon ground ginger

    ¼ teaspoon garlic powder

    ⅛ to ¼ teaspoon cayenne (optional)

Add enough water to the reserved pineapple juice to measure ½ cup. Put the pineapple and juice mixture in a small saucepan.

Stir in the pimiento and green onions. Bring to a simmer over medium-high heat. Stir in the rice. Reduce the heat and simmer, covered, for 10 minutes, or until the rice is tender and the liquid is absorbed.

Meanwhile, lightly spray the grill rack or broiler pan and rack with cooking spray. Preheat the grill on medium high or preheat the broiler.

Brush the oil over both sides of the fish.

In a small bowl, stir together the thyme, allspice, ginger, garlic powder, and cayenne. Sprinkle over both sides of the fish. Using your fingertips, gently press the mixture so it adheres to the fish.

Grill the fish, or broil it about 4 inches from the heat, for 3 to 5 minutes on each side, or until the desired doneness. Serve with the rice.

PER SERVING

Calories 254	Cholesterol 53 mg	DIETARY EXCHANGES:
Total Fat 5.0 g	Sodium 51 mg	1 starch
Saturated Fat 1.0 g	Carbohydrates 24 g	½ fruit
Trans Fat 0.0 g	Fiber 2 g	3 lean meat
Polyunsaturated Fat 1.0 g	Sugars 9 g	
Monounsaturated Fat 3.0 g	Protein 27 g	

Trout Amandine with Orange-Dijon Sauce

Serves 4

A perennial favorite, trout amandine, gets a modern makeover that includes a creamy yogurt sauce. Serve with Golden Rice (page 265) and your favorite green vegetable.

⅓ cup fat-free plain yogurt
1 tablespoon all-fruit orange marmalade
1 tablespoon Dijon mustard (lowest sodium available)
½ teaspoon salt-free lemon pepper
4 trout fillets with skin (about 4½ ounces each), rinsed and patted dry
3 tablespoons all-purpose flour
2 teaspoons olive oil
2 tablespoons sliced almonds

In a small bowl, whisk together the yogurt, marmalade, and mustard. Cover and refrigerate until needed.

Sprinkle the lemon pepper over the flesh side of the fish.

Put the flour in a medium shallow bowl. Dip the flesh side of the fish in the flour. Using your fingertips, gently press the flour so it adheres to the fish. Shake off any excess. Transfer to a plate.

Using a pastry brush, brush the oil over the flesh side of the fish. Sprinkle the almonds over the oil. Using your fingertips, gently press the almonds so they adhere to the fish.

Place the fish with the almond side down in a large nonstick skillet. Cook over medium-high heat for 3 to 4 minutes on each side, or until the fish flakes easily when tested with a fork.

Meanwhile, remove the sauce from the refrigerator if you want to serve it at room temperature rather than chilled.

Transfer the fish with the skin side up to a platter. Let cool for 1 minute. Using tongs, carefully peel off the skin. Turn so the almond-coated side faces up. Serve with the sauce.

COOK'S TIP ON TROUT: If your favorite seafood counter has only whole trout, look for one with clear eyes (not cloudy) and no fishy aroma. Ask for it to be "pan-dressed"—cleaned, trimmed, filleted, and ready to go in the pan.

PER SERVING

Calories 219
Total Fat 8.0 g
  Saturated Fat 1.5 g
  Trans Fat 0.0 g
  Polyunsaturated Fat 2.0 g
  Monounsaturated Fat 4.0 g

Cholesterol 67 mg
Sodium 128 mg
Carbohydrates 10 g
  Fiber 1 g
  Sugars 4 g
Protein 26 g

DIETARY EXCHANGES:
½ starch
3 lean meat

Mussels with Yogurt-Caper Sauce

Serves 6

A tangy yogurt dipping sauce seasoned with green onions, capers, and lemon complements the sweetness of tender mussels. Serve this distinctive dish with crusty whole-grain bread to soak up the fragrant cooking liquid, and a simple salad of dark, leafy greens dressed with Citrus-Tarragon Vinaigrette (page 102).

SAUCE

¾ cup fat-free plain yogurt

1 tablespoon finely chopped green onions (green part only)

1 tablespoon capers, drained

1 teaspoon grated lemon zest

¼ teaspoon sugar

. . . .

1 cup dry white wine (regular or nonalcoholic), dry vermouth, or water

1 small lemon, thinly sliced

2 tablespoons coarsely chopped fresh basil or 2 teaspoons dried basil, crumbled

2 medium garlic cloves, minced

1½ pounds fresh debearded and rinsed medium mussels in shells

In a small bowl, stir together the sauce ingredients. Cover and refrigerate until serving time.

In a stockpot, bring the remaining ingredients except the mussels to a boil over high heat. Stir in the mussels. Reduce the heat and simmer, covered, for 6 to 8 minutes, or until the shells open. Using tongs or a slotted spoon, discard any mussels that haven't opened. Transfer the mussels with the cooking liquid to a serving bowl. Serve the sauce on the side.

COOK'S TIP ON STORING GARLIC: Store fresh garlic at room temperature in a container or location that allows air circulation to prevent sprouting. It can last up to eight weeks.

COOK'S TIP ON FRESH MUSSELS: Use these rules of thumb when preparing fresh mussels: Be sure the mussels have no offensive odor, and don't use mussels with broken or cracked shells. If possible, cook mussels the day you buy them; don't wait longer than the next day. When choosing fresh mussels, look for those with closed shells. If the shell is open, give it a light tap to be sure it will close tightly. If it doesn't close, discard it. The reverse holds true once the mussels are cooked! The shells open if the mussels are fresh. Discard any mussels that don't open after cooking.

PER SERVING

Calories 147	Cholesterol 32 mg	DIETARY EXCHANGES:
Total Fat 2.5 g	Sodium 393 mg	½ other carbohydrate
Saturated Fat 0.5 g	Carbohydrates 8 g	2 lean meat
Trans Fat 0.0 g	Fiber 0 g	
Polyunsaturated Fat 0.5 g	Sugars 3 g	
Monounsaturated Fat 0.5 g	Protein 15 g	

Cajun Red Scallops

Serves 4

Creole or Cajun seasoning blend in its salt-free form is the perfect way to make the gentle flavor of scallops get up and dance. Watch the scallops carefully to keep them tender: As soon as they become opaque, remove them from the heat.

    6 ounces dried no-yolk noodles
    ½ teaspoon paprika
    ½ teaspoon salt-free Creole or Cajun seasoning blend
    1 pound sea scallops, rinsed and patted dry
    3 tablespoons light tub margarine
    1 teaspoon Dijon mustard (lowest sodium available)
    1 teaspoon grated lemon zest
    ¼ teaspoon salt
    1 teaspoon olive oil
    2 tablespoons finely chopped fresh parsley
    1 medium lemon, cut into 4 wedges

Prepare the noodles using the package directions, omitting the salt and margarine. Drain well in a colander. Transfer to a platter. Cover to keep warm.

Sprinkle the paprika and seasoning blend over the scallops.

In a small bowl, stir together the margarine, mustard, lemon zest, and salt.

In a large nonstick skillet, heat the oil over medium-high heat, swirling to coat the bottom. Cook the scallops for 3 minutes. Turn over the scallops. Cook for 2 minutes, or just until opaque in the center. Remove from the heat.

Using a rubber scraper, stir the margarine mixture into the scallops until completely blended, scraping the bottom and side of the skillet to dislodge any browned bits.

Spoon the scallops over the noodles. Sprinkle with the parsley. Serve with the lemon wedges.

....

COOK'S TIP ON JUICING CITRUS: If your lemon (or other citrus fruit) is hard or dry, microwave it at 100 percent power (high) for 20 to 30 seconds before juicing it to get a better yield.

....

COOK'S TIP ON CREOLE OR CAJUN SEASONING BLEND: To make your own salt-free Creole or Cajun seasoning blend, stir together ½ teaspoon each of chili powder, ground cumin, onion powder, garlic powder, paprika, and pepper, and, if you wish, ⅛ teaspoon of cayenne. This makes just over 1 tablespoon of the blend; double or triple the amounts if you like, and keep the extra in a container with a shaker top to use in other seafood, poultry, meat, and vegetable dishes.

PER SERVING

Calories 279	Cholesterol 27 mg	DIETARY EXCHANGES:
Total Fat 5.5 g	Sodium 560 mg	2½ starch
Saturated Fat 0.5 g	Carbohydrates 36 g	2 lean meat
Trans Fat 0.0 g	Fiber 2 g	
Polyunsaturated Fat 1.0 g	Sugars 2 g	
Monounsaturated Fat 3.0 g	Protein 19 g	

Seafood and Lemon Risotto

Serves 4

Creamy Arborio rice joins scallops and shrimp in this hearty entrée, made colorful by snow peas and red bell pepper. This recipe uses a preparation method that lets you stir less than most other risotto recipes.

Cooking spray

1 medium leek, sliced

2 medium garlic cloves, minced

1 cup uncooked Arborio rice

1½ cups fat-free, low-sodium chicken broth and ½ cup fat-free, low-sodium chicken broth, divided use

1 cup dry white wine (regular or nonalcoholic)

8 ounces peeled raw medium shrimp, rinsed and patted dry

8 ounces bay scallops, rinsed and patted dry

3 ounces snow peas, trimmed and halved

½ medium red bell pepper, chopped

3 tablespoons shredded or grated Parmesan cheese and 2 tablespoons shredded or grated Parmesan cheese, divided use

2 tablespoons chopped fresh basil or 2 teaspoons dried basil, crumbled

1½ to 2 tablespoons finely shredded lemon zest

Lightly spray a medium saucepan with cooking spray. Cook the leek and garlic over medium-low heat for 5 minutes, or until the leek is soft.

Stir in the rice. Cook for 5 minutes, stirring frequently.

Stir in 1½ cups broth. Increase the heat to high and bring to a boil, stirring occasionally. Reduce the heat and simmer for 5 minutes, stirring occasionally.

Pour in the remaining ½ cup broth and the wine. Increase the heat to medium and cook for 5 to 8 minutes, stirring constantly (a small amount of liquid should remain).

Stir the shrimp, scallops, peas, and bell pepper into the rice mixture. Cook for 5 minutes, or until the liquid is almost absorbed, stirring constantly. (The rice should be just tender and slightly creamy.)

Stir in 3 tablespoons Parmesan, the basil, and lemon zest.

Spoon the mixture onto plates. Sprinkle with the remaining 2 tablespoons Parmesan.

COOK'S TIP: For proper consistency, carefully regulate the cooking temperature so the risotto boils lightly, not vigorously. If the liquid is absorbed before the rice reaches the just-tender stage, add more broth, wine, or water, a little at a time. Arborio rice is usually used in risottos, but you can substitute a medium-grain rice if you prefer. It won't be quite as creamy, however.

PER SERVING

Calories 339	Cholesterol 109 mg	DIETARY EXCHANGES:
Total Fat 3.0 g	Sodium 434 mg	3 starch
Saturated Fat 1.0 g	Carbohydrates 47 g	1 vegetable
Trans Fat 0.0 g	Fiber 4 g	3 lean meat
Polyunsaturated Fat 0.5 g	Sugars 3 g	
Monounsaturated Fat 0.5 g	Protein 27 g	

Seared Tuna with Mango-Pear Salsa

Serves 4

The unexpected combination of mango and pear does delicious work as a salsa here. Chop the fruit into slightly larger pieces to transform the salsa into a salad to serve with other entrées, such as Asian Grilled Chicken (page 142) or Grilled Teriyaki Sirloin (page 182).

SALSA

- 1 medium mango, chopped
- ½ firm pear, peeled if desired and chopped
- 1 medium fresh jalapeño, seeds and ribs discarded, finely chopped (see Cook's Tip on page 101)
- 2 tablespoons finely chopped red onion
- 2 tablespoons chopped fresh cilantro
- ½ teaspoon grated lemon zest
- 1 tablespoon fresh lemon juice
- 1 to 2 teaspoons grated peeled gingerroot

. . . .

- 1 teaspoon chili powder
- ½ teaspoon pepper (coarsely ground preferred)
- ¼ teaspoon salt
- 4 tuna steaks (about 4 ounces each), about 1 inch thick, rinsed and patted dry
- 2 teaspoons canola or corn oil

In a medium bowl, gently stir together the salsa ingredients. Set aside.

In a small bowl, stir together the chili powder, pepper, and salt. Sprinkle the mixture over both sides of the fish. Using your fingertips, gently press the mixture so it adheres to the fish.

In a large nonstick skillet, heat the oil over medium-high heat, swirling to coat the bottom. Cook the fish for 4 minutes on each side, or until the desired doneness. Serve with the salsa.

PER SERVING

Calories 208	Cholesterol 53 mg	DIETARY EXCHANGES:
Total Fat 4.0 g	Sodium 200 mg	1 fruit
Saturated Fat 0.5 g	Carbohydrates 18 g	3 lean meat
Trans Fat 0.0 g	Fiber 3 g	
Polyunsaturated Fat 1.0 g	Sugars 14 g	
Monounsaturated Fat 2.0 g	Protein 26 g	

Poultry

ASIAN GRILLED CHICKEN 142

CRISPY OVEN-FRIED CHICKEN 144

GARLIC CHICKEN FILLETS IN BALSAMIC VINEGAR 145

CHICKEN BREASTS STUFFED WITH RICOTTA AND GOAT CHEESE 146

QUICK CURRY-BAKED CHICKEN WITH CUCUMBER RAITA 148

CHICKEN AND TORTILLA CASSEROLE 150

CHICKEN WITH MUSHROOM-SHERRY SAUCE 152

CHICKEN WITH SPICY BLACK PEPPER SAUCE 153

CHICKEN FAJITAS 154

CHICKEN SOUTHWESTERN 156

CREAMY CHICKEN CURRY 158

CHINESE-STYLE CHICKEN AND SOBA NOODLES 160

SLOW-COOKER TUSCAN CHICKEN 162

BRUNSWICK STEW 163

MOROCCAN CHICKEN 164

CAJUN CHICKEN PASTA 165

THAI CHICKEN WITH BASIL AND VEGETABLES 166

GREEK-STYLE STEWED CHICKEN 168

CHICKEN AND VEGGIE BAKE 169

CHICKEN AND VEGETABLE LASAGNA 170

CHICKEN POT PIE WITH MASHED POTATO TOPPING 172

CUMIN-ROASTED TURKEY BREAST WITH RASPBERRY SAUCE 174

TURKEY MEATBALLS IN SQUASH SHELLS 176

TURKEY PATTIES WITH FRESH BASIL-MUSHROOM SAUCE 178

Asian Grilled Chicken

Serves 6

The sweet and tart marinade is delicious, but it does need some time to impart its flavor, so prepare this on an evening when you're not too rushed. For a super-simple side, try Sweet-and-Sour Broccoli and Red Bell Pepper (page 251), which also needs some marinating time.

MARINADE

- ¼ cup soy sauce (lowest sodium available)
- ¼ cup honey
- 3 tablespoons red wine vinegar
- 2 tablespoons finely chopped fresh parsley
- 2 teaspoons grated peeled gingerroot or 1 teaspoon ground ginger
- ½ teaspoon pepper
- 1 medium garlic clove, minced
  . . . .
- 3 skinless chicken breasts with bone (about 12 ounces each), all visible fat discarded
  Cooking spray

In a small nonmetallic bowl, whisk together the marinade ingredients. Pour ½ cup of the marinade into a large shallow dish. Add the chicken to the marinade in the dish, turning to coat. Cover and refrigerate for at least 2 hours, turning occasionally. Cover and refrigerate the marinade in the small bowl until needed.

When the chicken has marinated, lightly spray a grill rack with cooking spray. Preheat the grill on high.

Drain the chicken, discarding the marinade in the dish. Grill the chicken for 30 to 45 minutes, or until no longer pink in the center, brushing with the reserved marinade in the bowl and turning frequently. To protect against harmful bacteria, be sure to wash the basting brush between basting steps until the chicken surface turns white. (Washing the brush isn't necessary after this point.) Cut each breast in half before serving.

COOK'S TIP: To broil the chicken, follow the instructions above except preheat the broiler and lightly spray a broiler-safe baking sheet with cooking spray. Broil about 5 inches from the heat for 25 to 30 minutes, basting as directed.

COOK'S TIP ON SKINNING POULTRY: You can dramatically reduce the amount of saturated fat in poultry by discarding the skin. Because of its slippery nature, poultry skin can be a challenge to remove, however. Hold a piece of poultry on a flat surface (a plastic cutting board is recommended), grasp the skin with a double thickness of paper towels, and pull firmly. Discard the skin and the paper towels. Use a knife or kitchen scissors to trim any remaining visible fat.

PER SERVING

Calories 172	Cholesterol 87 mg	DIETARY EXCHANGES:
Total Fat 3.5 g	Sodium 418 mg	½ other carbohydrate
Saturated Fat 1.0 g	Carbohydrates 4 g	4 lean meat
Trans Fat 0.0 g	Fiber 0 g	
Polyunsaturated Fat 0.5 g	Sugars 4 g	
Monounsaturated Fat 1.0 g	Protein 30 g	

Crispy Oven-Fried Chicken

Serves 6

This spicy, heart-friendly alternative to traditional fried chicken surprises your taste buds with a pleasant nip of ginger. Try it with Individual Corn Puddings (page 259), which bake at the same temperature, or with Sautéed Greens and Cabbage (page 261).

Cooking spray (butter flavor preferred)
1 teaspoon ground ginger, or to taste
1 teaspoon paprika
¼ teaspoon salt
Pepper to taste
3 skinless chicken breasts with bone (about 12 ounces each), all visible fat discarded
4 cups wheat-flake or cornflake cereal, lightly crushed
1 medium garlic clove, crushed (optional)

Preheat the oven to 350°F. Lightly spray a baking sheet with cooking spray.

In a small bowl, stir together the ginger, paprika, salt, and pepper. Sprinkle over both sides of the chicken.

In a pie pan, stir together the cereal and garlic. Dip the chicken in the mixture, turning to coat and gently shaking off any excess. Using your fingertips, gently press the coating so it adheres to the chicken.

Lightly spray the chicken on all sides with cooking spray. Transfer to the baking sheet.

Bake for 45 minutes to 1 hour, or until the chicken is golden brown, tender, and no longer pink in the center. (The timing depends on the thickness of the chicken.) Cut each breast in half before serving.

PER SERVING

Calories 241	Cholesterol 87 mg	DIETARY EXCHANGES:
Total Fat 4.0 g	Sodium 358 mg	1½ starch
Saturated Fat 1.0 g	Carbohydrates 20 g	4 lean meat
Trans Fat 0.0 g	Fiber 3 g	
Polyunsaturated Fat 1.0 g	Sugars 4 g	
Monounsaturated Fat 1.0 g	Protein 31 g	

Garlic Chicken Fillets in Balsamic Vinegar

Serves 8

The dark sweetness of balsamic vinegar, which is produced in two regions in northern Italy, gently blankets chicken fillets sprinkled with garlic in this sophisticated, Italian-inspired dish.

8 boneless, skinless chicken breast halves (about 4 ounces each), all visible fat discarded
½ cup all-purpose flour
2 teaspoons olive oil
Cooking spray
6 to 8 medium garlic cloves, minced
1 cup fat-free, low-sodium chicken broth
⅓ cup balsamic vinegar
Pepper to taste
1 tablespoon cornstarch
2 tablespoons water

Put the chicken on a plate. Sprinkle the flour over both sides of the chicken, shaking off any excess.

In a large nonstick skillet, heat the oil over medium-high heat, swirling to coat the bottom. Cook the chicken for 2 to 3 minutes, or until the bottom is golden. Lightly spray the top with cooking spray. Turn over the chicken. Sprinkle with the garlic. Cook for 2 to 3 minutes, or until golden.

Add the broth, vinegar, and pepper. Reduce the heat to medium low. Cook, covered, for 5 to 10 minutes, or until the chicken is tender and no longer pink in the center. Leaving the liquid in the skillet, transfer the chicken to a platter. Cover to keep warm.

Put the cornstarch in a small bowl. Add the water, whisking to dissolve. Pour into the skillet. Increase the heat to high and bring to a boil. Boil for 1 to 2 minutes, or until the liquid is thick and smooth, whisking occasionally. Pour over the chicken.

PER SERVING

Calories 186	Cholesterol 73 mg	DIETARY EXCHANGES:
Total Fat 4.0 g	Sodium 142 mg	½ starch
Saturated Fat 1.0 g	Carbohydrates 10 g	3 lean meat
Trans Fat 0.0 g	Fiber 0 g	
Polyunsaturated Fat 0.5 g	Sugars 2 g	
Monounsaturated Fat 1.5 g	Protein 25 g	

Chicken Breasts Stuffed with Ricotta and Goat Cheese

Serves 4

With its creamy stuffing and herbed sauce, this chicken dish will rise to even the most august occasion. Happily, it's a snap to make and the tomato sauce keeps the chicken moist. Wilted Spinach (page 268) makes an equally impressive side dish.

Cooking spray

STUFFING

7 ounces fat-free ricotta cheese

2 ounces soft goat cheese

2 tablespoons chopped fresh parsley or 2 teaspoons dried parsley, crumbled

1 tablespoon finely chopped green onions (green part only)

SAUCE

1 8-ounce can no-salt-added tomato sauce

2 teaspoons dried Italian seasoning, crumbled

1½ teaspoons chopped fresh oregano or ½ teaspoon dried oregano, crumbled

1 medium garlic clove, minced

¼ teaspoon salt

⅛ teaspoon pepper

. . . .

4 boneless, skinless chicken breast halves (about 4 ounces each), all visible fat discarded, flattened to ¼-inch thickness

Preheat the oven to 350°F. Lightly spray an 8-inch square glass baking dish with cooking spray.

In a small bowl, stir together the stuffing ingredients.

In a separate small bowl, stir together the sauce ingredients.

Spoon about one-fourth of the stuffing down the center of each chicken breast. Starting with the short end, roll up jelly-roll style. Place with the seam side down in the dish. Spoon the sauce over the chicken.

Bake, covered, for 40 to 45 minutes, or until the chicken is no longer pink in the center.

....

COOK'S TIP ON GREEN ONIONS: Many recipes call for only the dark green parts of the green onion. Cut off the green tops to about 3 inches above the white bulbs, and set the green onions in a glass, root end down. Add about 2 inches of water. Place the glass on a sunny windowsill and change the water daily. You'll have new green tops in about a week.

....

PER SERVING

Calories 222	Cholesterol 83 mg	DIETARY EXCHANGES:
Total Fat 6.0 g	Sodium 433 mg	1 vegetable
Saturated Fat 2.5 g	Carbohydrates 6 g	4 lean meat
Trans Fat 0.0 g	Fiber 1 g	
Polyunsaturated Fat 0.5 g	Sugars 4 g	
Monounsaturated Fat 1.5 g	Protein 34 g	

Quick Curry-Baked Chicken with Cucumber Raita

Serves 4

In a hurry but tired of the same old go-to chicken dish? This curried version kicks dinner up a notch and is complemented by a cool and refreshing cucumber raita (RI-tah), an Indian yogurt sauce. Try this entrée over quick-and-easy whole-grain couscous.

    Cooking spray
1 teaspoon curry powder
½ teaspoon ground cumin
¼ teaspoon onion powder or garlic powder
⅛ teaspoon cayenne
4 boneless, skinless chicken breast halves (about 4 ounces each), all visible fat discarded

RAITA

1 small cucumber, peeled, halved lengthwise, and seeds discarded
⅛ teaspoon salt
8 ounces fat-free plain yogurt
¼ cup finely diced red bell pepper
2 tablespoons finely chopped fresh parsley or cilantro
½ teaspoon grated peeled gingerroot
¼ teaspoon cumin seeds or ground cumin
    Pepper to taste

Preheat the oven to 350°F. Lightly spray a baking sheet with cooking spray.

In a small bowl, stir together the curry powder, cumin, onion powder, and cayenne. Sprinkle over both sides of the chicken. Place the chicken with the smooth side up on the baking sheet. Lightly spray the chicken with cooking spray.

Bake for 20 minutes, or until the chicken is no longer pink in the center.

Meanwhile, grate the cucumber. Transfer to a colander and sprinkle with the salt. Let drain for at least 5 minutes. Squeeze the cucumber to remove the excess liquid. Pat dry with paper towels.

In a medium serving bowl, thoroughly whisk the yogurt. Stir in the cucumber and the remaining raita ingredients except the pepper. Cover and refrigerate until the chicken is done. Just before serving, sprinkle the raita with the pepper. Serve with the chicken.

PER SERVING

Calories 173	Cholesterol 74 mg	DIETARY EXCHANGES:
Total Fat 3.5 g	Sodium 251 mg	½ fat-free milk
Saturated Fat 0.5 g	Carbohydrates 7 g	3 lean meat
Trans Fat 0.0 g	Fiber 1 g	
Polyunsaturated Fat 0.5 g	Sugars 5 g	
Monounsaturated Fat 1.0 g	Protein 28 g	

Chicken and Tortilla Casserole

Serves 8

This dish tastes somewhat like chicken enchiladas but is prepared without all the fuss. The green tomatillo sauce (or salsa verde) in this recipe can be used over enchiladas, chicken, or fish, or even as a dip for baked, unsalted tortilla chips.

Cooking spray
10 **6-inch corn tortillas**
1 **teaspoon canola or corn oil**
1 **medium onion, chopped**
2 **medium garlic cloves, minced**
2 **cups fat-free, low-sodium chicken broth**
1 **12-ounce can no-salt-added tomatillos, drained**
1 **medium fresh jalapeño, seeds and ribs discarded (see Cook's Tip on page 101)**
⅛ **teaspoon pepper**
2 **pounds boneless, skinless chicken breasts, cooked without salt, all visible fat discarded, cubed**
1 **cup shredded low-fat Monterey Jack cheese**
½ **cup fat-free sour cream**

Preheat the oven to 350°F. Lightly spray a 13 x 9 x 2-inch baking dish with cooking spray.

Cut the tortillas into quarters and arrange in a single layer on a large ungreased baking sheet. Bake for 10 minutes, or until crisp. Set aside.

In a large skillet, heat the oil over medium heat, swirling to coat the bottom. Cook the onion and garlic for 2 to 3 minutes, or until the onion is almost soft, stirring frequently.

In a food processor or blender, process the broth, tomatillos, jalapeño, and pepper until smooth. Stir into the onion mixture. Bring to a simmer and simmer for 15 minutes.

In the baking dish, arrange the layers as follows: half the tortilla quarters, half the chicken, half the tomatillo mixture, and half the Monterey Jack. Repeat the layers.

Bake for 40 minutes. Remove from the oven.

Spread the sour cream over the top of the casserole. Serve warm.

COOK'S TIP: It's so convenient to cook extra chicken breasts to keep in the freezer for those hectic nights, but if you don't have any available for this dish, discard all the visible fat from 2 pounds of skinless, boneless chicken breasts, then cut the chicken into bite-size cubes. Lightly spray a large skillet with cooking spray. Heat over medium-high heat. Cook the chicken for 3 to 4 minutes, or until no longer pink in the center, stirring constantly.

PER SERVING

Calories 232	Cholesterol 78 mg	DIETARY EXCHANGES:
Total Fat 5.0 g	Sodium 271 mg	½ starch
Saturated Fat 1.5 g	Carbohydrates 15 g	1 vegetable
Trans Fat 0.0 g	Fiber 2 g	3½ lean meat
Polyunsaturated Fat 1.0 g	Sugars 4 g	
Monounsaturated Fat 1.5 g	Protein 31 g	

Chicken with Mushroom-Sherry Sauce

Serves 4

Stirring in the final spoons of dry sherry after reducing the sauce gives it exhilarating warmth. Choose Apple-Lemon Carrots (page 255) for a brightly colored side with a delicate citrus flavor.

¼ teaspoon salt and ¼ teaspoon salt, divided use
¼ teaspoon pepper
4 boneless, skinless chicken breast halves (about 4 ounces each), all visible fat discarded
1 tablespoon olive oil
8 ounces sliced button mushrooms
1 medium onion, thinly sliced
¼ teaspoon dried thyme, crumbled
⅓ cup dry sherry or 100% apple cider and 2 tablespoons plus 2 teaspoons dry sherry or 100% apple cider, divided use

Sprinkle ¼ teaspoon salt and the pepper over both sides of the chicken.

In a large nonstick skillet, heat the oil over medium heat, swirling to coat the bottom. Cook the chicken with the smooth side down for 4 minutes. Turn over the chicken. Cook for 2 to 4 minutes, or until no longer pink in the center. Transfer to a platter. Cover to keep warm.

In the same skillet, stir together the remaining ingredients except the sherry. Cook for 4 minutes, or until the onion is soft, stirring frequently.

Stir in ⅓ cup sherry. Increase the heat to high and bring to a boil. Boil for 1 minute, or until the liquid has almost evaporated, stirring occasionally. Remove from the heat.

Stir in the remaining 2 tablespoons plus 2 teaspoons sherry. Spoon the sauce over the chicken.

PER SERVING

Calories 204	Cholesterol 73 mg	DIETARY EXCHANGES:
Total Fat 6.5 g	Sodium 429 mg	1 vegetable
Saturated Fat 1.0 g	Carbohydrates 5 g	3 lean meat
Trans Fat 0.0 g	Fiber 1 g	
Polyunsaturated Fat 1.0 g	Sugars 3 g	
Monounsaturated Fat 3.5 g	Protein 26 g	

Chicken with Spicy Black Pepper Sauce

Serves 4

Liven up dinner with this triple-sauced poultry entrée. Serve it with a side that will help your palate mellow, such as Cucumber-Melon Salad with Raspberry Vinegar (page 75).

½ teaspoon pepper (coarsely ground preferred)
¼ teaspoon garlic powder
⅛ teaspoon salt
4 boneless, skinless chicken breast halves (about 4 ounces each), all visible fat discarded
1 teaspoon olive oil and 1 tablespoon olive oil, divided use
1 tablespoon soy sauce (lowest sodium available)
1 tablespoon steak sauce (lowest sodium available)
1 tablespoon Worcestershire sauce (lowest sodium available)
2 teaspoons fresh lime juice
1 medium Italian plum (Roma) tomato, finely chopped (optional)

In a small bowl, stir together the pepper, garlic powder, and salt. Sprinkle over both sides of the chicken. Using your fingertips, gently press the mixture so it adheres to the chicken.

In a large nonstick skillet, heat 1 teaspoon oil over medium heat, swirling to coat the bottom. Cook the chicken with the smooth side down for 4 minutes. Turn over the chicken. Cook for 2 to 4 minutes, or until no longer pink in the center. Transfer to plates.

In the same skillet, stir together the soy sauce, steak sauce, Worcestershire sauce, lime juice, and the remaining 1 tablespoon oil. Increase the heat to medium high and bring just to a boil, scraping the bottom and side of the skillet to dislodge any browned bits. Remove from the heat.

Spoon the sauce over the chicken. Sprinkle with the tomato.

PER SERVING

Calories 181	Cholesterol 73 mg	DIETARY EXCHANGES:
Total Fat 7.5 g	Sodium 342 mg	3 lean meat
Saturated Fat 1.5 g	Carbohydrates 3 g	
Trans Fat 0.0 g	Fiber 0 g	
Polyunsaturated Fat 1.0 g	Sugars 2 g	
Monounsaturated Fat 4.0 g	Protein 24 g	

Chicken Fajitas

Serves 4

Warm corn tortillas rolled around sizzling chicken, onion, and bell pepper will satisfy your craving for Mexican food in a healthy way. Shredded lettuce, chopped tomatoes, low-sodium salsa, and a dollop of fat-free sour cream are common accompaniments if you'd like to dress up these fajitas. For another level of flavor, drizzle on some Tomatillo-Avocado Dressing (page 101).

MARINADE

- 3 tablespoons Worcestershire sauce (lowest sodium available)
- 1½ tablespoons fresh lemon or lime juice
- 1 tablespoon water
- 1 teaspoon canola or corn oil
- 1 medium garlic clove, minced
- ½ teaspoon pepper, or to taste
  . . . .
- 1 pound boneless, skinless chicken breasts, all visible fat discarded, cut into ⅜-inch strips
- 1 large onion, cut into ⅛-inch strips
- 1 large green bell pepper, cut into ⅛-inch strips
- 1 teaspoon canola or corn oil and 1 teaspoon canola or corn oil, divided use
- 8 6-inch corn tortillas
- Cooking spray

In a large shallow dish, whisk together the marinade ingredients. Add the chicken to the marinade, turning to coat. Cover and refrigerate for 10 to 20 minutes, turning once halfway through.

Meanwhile, preheat the oven to 350°F.

Put the onion and bell pepper in a small bowl. Stir in 1 teaspoon oil.

When the chicken has marinated, wrap the tortillas in aluminum foil and heat in the oven for 8 to 10 minutes.

Meanwhile, lightly spray a large skillet with cooking spray. Pour in the remaining 1 teaspoon oil, swirling to coat the bottom. Heat over medium-high heat. Drain the chicken, discarding the marinade. Cook the chicken for 4 minutes, stirring occasionally.

Stir in the onion and bell pepper. Cook for 5 minutes, or until the onion is slightly browned and the chicken is no longer pink in the center, stirring constantly.

Spoon the chicken mixture onto the tortillas. Roll the tortillas around the filling, jelly-roll style.

PER SERVING

Calories 253	Cholesterol 73 mg	DIETARY EXCHANGES:
Total Fat 6.0 g	Sodium 231 mg	1 starch
Saturated Fat 1.0 g	Carbohydrates 22 g	1 vegetable
Trans Fat 0.0 g	Fiber 3 g	3 lean meat
Polyunsaturated Fat 1.5 g	Sugars 7 g	
Monounsaturated Fat 2.5 g	Protein 27 g	

Chicken Southwestern

Serves 6

Start your evening with Southwestern Black Bean Spread (page 35) and some baked unsalted corn tortilla chips for dipping. Serve this colorful and filling entrée, which has strong accents of chili powder and lime zest, as the centerpiece of your meal, and pair it with Jícama and Grapefruit Salad with Ancho-Honey Dressing (page 80), and Mango Brûlée with Pine Nuts (page 310) as a sweet finish.

- 1 tablespoon canola or corn oil and 2 tablespoons canola or corn oil, divided use
- 1½ cups orange, red, or yellow bell pepper strips
- 2 teaspoons minced fresh jalapeño, seeds and ribs discarded (see Cook's Tip on page 101)
- 4 medium green onions, sliced diagonally
- ⅓ cup all-purpose flour
- 1½ teaspoons chili powder and 2 teaspoons chili powder, divided use
- ¼ teaspoon pepper and ½ teaspoon pepper (freshly ground preferred), divided use
- ¼ teaspoon salt
- 1½ pounds chicken breast halves, all visible fat discarded, flattened to ⅛-inch thickness
- 1 28-ounce can no-salt-added whole tomatoes, undrained
- 1½ teaspoons grated lime zest

In a large nonstick skillet, heat 1 tablespoon oil over medium-high heat, swirling to coat the bottom. Cook the bell pepper and jalapeño for 4 to 5 minutes, stirring frequently. Stir in the green onions. Cook for 1 minute. Transfer the mixture to a large plate. Set aside.

In a medium shallow dish, stir together the flour, 1½ teaspoons chili powder, ¼ teaspoon pepper, and the salt. Dip the chicken in the flour mixture, turning to coat and gently shaking off any excess. Transfer the chicken to a separate plate.

In the same skillet, still over medium-high heat, heat the remaining 2 tablespoons oil, swirling to coat the bottom. Cook half the chicken for 3 minutes, or until lightly browned on both sides, turning once halfway through (the chicken won't be done at this point). Transfer to the large plate with the bell pepper mixture. Repeat with the remaining chicken.

Put the tomatoes with liquid in the skillet. Using a wooden spoon, gently break up the tomatoes. Stir in the remaining 2 teaspoons chili powder and ½ teaspoon pepper. Cook over medium-high heat for 3 to 4 minutes, stirring occasionally.

Stir in the lime zest, bell pepper mixture, and chicken. Cook for 3 minutes, or until the chicken is no longer pink in the center.

PER SERVING

Calories 272	Cholesterol 73 mg	DIETARY EXCHANGES:
Total Fat 10.5 g	Sodium 275 mg	½ starch
Saturated Fat 1.0 g	Carbohydrates 16 g	2 vegetable
Trans Fat 0.0 g	Fiber 3 g	3 lean meat
Polyunsaturated Fat 2.5 g	Sugars 6 g	
Monounsaturated Fat 5.5 g	Protein 27 g	

Creamy Chicken Curry

Serves 6

This intricately flavored dish brings the warmth and intensity of Indian cuisine to your table. Serve over basmati rice so you can savor all the deep orange sauce, speckled with vibrant green cilantro.

- 2 tablespoons canola or corn oil
- 1 medium onion, finely chopped
- 2 teaspoons garlic powder
- 1 6-ounce can no-salt-added tomato paste
- 2 teaspoons ground cumin
- 1½ teaspoons ground coriander
- ½ teaspoon ground turmeric
- ½ teaspoon cayenne
- 1 pound boneless, skinless chicken breasts, all visible fat discarded, cut into bite-size pieces
- 1 cup fat-free sour cream
- ½ teaspoon salt
- 1 medium fresh jalapeño, seeds and ribs discarded, chopped (see Cook's Tip on page 101)
- 1 tablespoon minced peeled gingerroot
- ½ cup finely chopped fresh cilantro
- 1 teaspoon garam masala (optional)

In a large skillet, heat the oil over medium-high heat, swirling to coat the bottom. Cook the onion for about 3 minutes, or until soft, stirring frequently.

Stir in the garlic powder. Cook for 1 minute, stirring constantly.

Stir in the tomato paste, cumin, coriander, turmeric, and cayenne. Cook for 1 minute, stirring occasionally.

Stir in the chicken, sour cream, and salt. If the mixture seems dry, gradually stir in a little water as needed. Bring to a boil. Reduce the heat and simmer for 15 minutes, stirring occasionally.

Stir in the jalapeño and gingerroot. Cook for 10 minutes, or until the chicken is no longer pink in the center.

Just before serving, sprinkle with the cilantro and garam masala.

COOK'S TIP ON GARAM MASALA: Dry-roasted spices are ground together to make the distinctive blend known as garam masala. It may include 10 to 12 different spices, such as cumin, coriander, cloves, cardamom, black pepper, and mace, and is usually added to food near the end of cooking or right before the dish is served to enhance the complexity of flavor.

PER SERVING

Calories 208	Cholesterol 55 mg	DIETARY EXCHANGES:
Total Fat 7.0 g	Sodium 335 mg	½ starch
Saturated Fat 1.0 g	Carbohydrates 16 g	2 vegetable
Trans Fat 0.0 g	Fiber 2 g	2½ lean meat
Polyunsaturated Fat 1.5 g	Sugars 8 g	
Monounsaturated Fat 3.5 g	Protein 21 g	

Chinese-Style Chicken and Soba Noodles

Serves 6

Forget Chinese takeout tonight and stay in to enjoy this spicy dish, which is teeming with a variety of vegetables and bites of juicy mango. And it's cooked in a slow cooker, so it takes just a few minutes of hands-on time.

1½ pounds boneless, skinless chicken breasts, all visible fat discarded, cut into bite-size pieces

1 8-ounce can sliced water chestnuts, drained

8 ounces button mushrooms, sliced

2 stalks of baby bok choy (about 6 ounces total), stems and leaves cut crosswise into ¼-inch slices (about 1½ cups sliced)

2 medium carrots, cut into ¼-inch slices

1 cup chopped onion

¾ cup sweet-and-sour sauce (lowest sodium available)

2 teaspoons grated peeled gingerroot

2 teaspoons soy sauce (lowest sodium available)

1 teaspoon crushed red pepper flakes

1 teaspoon toasted sesame oil

½ teaspoon garlic powder

. . . .

1 large mango, cut into bite-size pieces

2 tablespoons cornstarch

2 tablespoons water

6 ounces dried soba noodles

In a 4- to 5-quart round or oval slow cooker, stir together the chicken, water chestnuts, mushrooms, bok choy, carrots, and onion.

In a small bowl, whisk together the sweet-and-sour sauce, gingerroot, soy sauce, red pepper flakes, sesame oil, and garlic powder. Pour over the chicken mixture, stirring to combine. Cook, covered, on low for 7 to 8 hours or on high for 3½ to 4 hours.

Stir the mango into the chicken mixture. Put the cornstarch in a small bowl. Add the water, whisking to dissolve. Stir into the chicken mixture. If using the low setting, change it to high. Cook, covered, for 10 to 15 minutes, or until the sauce is slightly thickened.

Meanwhile, prepare the soba noodles using the package directions, omitting the salt. Serve the chicken mixture over the noodles.

....

COOK'S TIP ON CUTTING MANGOES: To cut a mango, place it on its side on a cutting board. Cutting downward, slice off each side of the mango, avoiding the large seed in the middle. Slice off the top and the bottom. Peel and slice or chop as desired.

....

PER SERVING

Calories 376	Cholesterol 73 mg	DIETARY EXCHANGES:
Total Fat 4.5 g	Sodium 264 mg	2 starch
Saturated Fat 1.0 g	Carbohydrates 54 g	1 fruit
Trans Fat 0.0 g	Fiber 5 g	2 vegetable
Polyunsaturated Fat 1.0 g	Sugars 24 g	3 lean meat
Monounsaturated Fat 1.5 g	Protein 31 g	

Slow-Cooker Tuscan Chicken

Serves 8

This easy, sunny-tasting chicken dish showcases ingredients often used in Tuscan cooking, such as artichokes and black olives. Try it over farro or whole-grain pasta.

- 1 **teaspoon dried basil, crumbled**
- 1 **teaspoon dried oregano, crumbled**
- 2 **pounds boneless, skinless chicken breasts, all visible fat discarded**
- 1 **14.5-ounce can no-salt-added diced tomatoes, undrained**
- 9 **ounces frozen artichoke hearts, thawed**
- 1 **cup fat-free, low-sodium chicken broth**
- 1 **2.25-ounce can sliced black olives, drained**
- ¼ **teaspoon salt**
- ¼ **teaspoon pepper**
- ¼ **teaspoon crushed red pepper flakes (optional)**

Sprinkle the basil and oregano over both sides of the chicken. Put the chicken in a 3½- to 4-quart round or oval slow cooker.

Stir in the remaining ingredients, including the tomatoes with liquid. Cook, covered, on low for 7 to 8 hours or on high for 3 to 4 hours.

PER SERVING

Calories 166	Cholesterol 73 mg	DIETARY EXCHANGES:
Total Fat 4.0 g	Sodium 308 mg	1 vegetable
Saturated Fat 1.0 g	Carbohydrates 6 g	3 lean meat
Trans Fat 0.0 g	Fiber 4 g	
Polyunsaturated Fat 0.5 g	Sugars 2 g	
Monounsaturated Fat 1.5 g	Protein 26 g	

Brunswick Stew

Serves 6

Brimming with vegetables and tender cubes of chicken, this well-known stew from Brunswick County in central Virginia will warm you from head to toe on a cold, snowy day. The original recipe dates back to 1828 and was served for dinner on hunting trips. Many cooks have created many delicious variations since that time, and this one is no exception.

Cooking spray
1 teaspoon olive oil
1 medium onion, chopped
1 pound boneless, skinless chicken breasts, all visible fat discarded, cut into 1-inch cubes
3 cups fat-free, low-sodium chicken broth
2 cups fresh or frozen whole-kernel corn
1½ cups fresh or frozen baby lima beans
1½ cups chopped tomatoes
1 6-ounce can no-salt-added tomato paste
3 tablespoons fresh lemon juice
1 tablespoon Worcestershire sauce (lowest sodium available)

Lightly spray a large, deep skillet or Dutch oven with cooking spray. Pour in the oil, swirling to coat the bottom. Heat over medium-high heat. Cook the onion for 3 minutes, or until soft, stirring frequently.

Stir in the remaining ingredients. Reduce the heat and simmer, covered, for 1 hour.

PER SERVING		
Calories 238	Cholesterol 48 mg	DIETARY EXCHANGES:
Total Fat 3.5 g	Sodium 276 mg	1½ starch
Saturated Fat 0.5 g	Carbohydrates 29 g	2 vegetable
Trans Fat 0.0 g	Fiber 6 g	2½ lean meat
Polyunsaturated Fat 0.5 g	Sugars 11 g	
Monounsaturated Fat 1.5 g	Protein 23 g	

Moroccan Chicken

Serves 4

The power of spice is beautifully demonstrated in this classic dish with Moroccan influences. Fluffy couscous absorbs and distributes the flavors. Serve with steamed spinach, roasted cauliflower, or Roasted Brussels Sprouts (page 252).

2 teaspoons olive oil
1 pound boneless, skinless chicken breasts, all visible fat discarded, each breast quartered
1 medium onion, cut into eighths
4 medium garlic cloves, minced
¾ cup fat-free, low-sodium chicken broth
½ cup dry white wine (regular or nonalcoholic) or water
¼ cup kalamata olives, coarsely chopped
1 medium lemon, cut into 4 wedges
1 teaspoon grated peeled gingerroot
½ teaspoon paprika
¼ teaspoon ground turmeric
⅛ teaspoon pepper
¾ cup uncooked whole-wheat couscous
⅛ teaspoon salt

In a large nonstick skillet, heat the oil over medium-high heat, swirling to coat the bottom. Cook the chicken for 2 minutes on each side, or until lightly browned. Stir in the onion and garlic. Cook for 4 to 5 minutes, or until the onion is tender-crisp, stirring occasionally.

Stir in the broth, wine, olives, lemon wedges, gingerroot, paprika, turmeric, and pepper. Bring to a boil, stirring occasionally. Reduce the heat and simmer, covered, for 15 to 20 minutes, or until the chicken is no longer pink in the center. Stir in the couscous and salt. Remove from the heat.

Let stand, covered, for 5 minutes, or until the liquid is absorbed and the couscous is tender. (Don't stir while the mixture stands.) Fluff with a fork. Discard the lemon wedges.

PER SERVING

Calories 376	Cholesterol 73 mg	DIETARY EXCHANGES:
Total Fat 9.0 g	Sodium 392 mg	2½ starch
Saturated Fat 1.5 g	Carbohydrates 39 g	1 vegetable
Trans Fat 0.0 g	Fiber 6 g	3 lean meat
Polyunsaturated Fat 1.5 g	Sugars 2 g	
Monounsaturated Fat 5.0 g	Protein 31 g	

Cajun Chicken Pasta

Serves 4

Tender twists of gemelli pasta, browned chicken, and a creamy, moderately spicy sauce make this combination hard to resist.

8 ounces dried whole-grain pasta, such as gemelli, rotini, or penne

1 teaspoon canola or corn oil

1 pound chicken breast tenders, all visible fat discarded

1½ teaspoons salt-free Creole or Cajun seasoning blend

1 medium green bell pepper, chopped

1 medium onion, chopped

2 medium ribs of celery, chopped

2 medium garlic cloves, minced

1½ cups fat-free, low-sodium chicken broth

2 tablespoons all-purpose flour

½ cup fat-free half-and-half

¼ teaspoon salt

Prepare the pasta using the package directions, omitting the salt. Drain well in a colander. Set aside.

Meanwhile, in a large nonstick skillet, heat the oil over medium-high heat, swirling to coat the bottom. Put the chicken in the skillet. Sprinkle the seasoning blend over the chicken. Cook the chicken for 2 minutes on each side, or until browned.

Stir in the bell pepper, onion, celery, and garlic. Cook for 2 to 3 minutes, or until the vegetables are tender-crisp, stirring occasionally.

Pour in the broth. Bring to a simmer. Reduce the heat and simmer, covered, for 8 to 10 minutes, or until the vegetables are tender and the chicken is no longer pink in the center.

Put the flour in a small bowl. Pour in the half-and-half, whisking until smooth. Stir into the chicken mixture. Increase the heat to medium high and cook for 3 to 4 minutes, or until the sauce is thickened, stirring occasionally.

Stir in the pasta and salt. Cook for 2 to 3 minutes, or until heated through.

PER SERVING

Calories 403	Cholesterol 73 mg	DIETARY EXCHANGES:
Total Fat 6.0 g	Sodium 348 mg	3 starch
Saturated Fat 1.0 g	Carbohydrates 54 g	2 vegetable
Trans Fat 0.0 g	Fiber 8 g	3 lean meat
Polyunsaturated Fat 1.5 g	Sugars 7 g	
Monounsaturated Fat 2.0 g	Protein 35 g	

Thai Chicken with Basil and Vegetables

Serves 4

Undertones of Thai basil, which has a licoricelike and spicy flavor, underscore the natural flavors of chicken, broccoli, carrots, and green onions in this all-in-one meal. Because this dish cooks quickly, have your ingredients gathered and prepped before you start stir-frying.

1   **cup uncooked rice (brown or jasmine preferred)**

SAUCE

2   **tablespoons fat-free, low-sodium chicken broth or water**
2   **teaspoons sugar**
2   **teaspoons fish sauce (lowest sodium available)**
1   **teaspoon soy sauce (lowest sodium available)**
. . . .

1   **teaspoon canola or corn oil**
2   **medium garlic cloves, minced**
1   **serrano pepper, seeds and ribs discarded, chopped (optional) (see Cook's Tip on page 101)**
1   **pound boneless, skinless chicken breasts, all visible fat discarded, cut into thin slices**
2   **cups broccoli florets**
2   **medium carrots, cut into matchstick-size strips**
4   **medium green onions, cut into 1-inch pieces**
¼   **cup tightly packed fresh Thai basil, sliced**

Prepare the rice using the package directions, omitting the salt and margarine. Set aside.

In a small bowl, whisk together the sauce ingredients. Set aside.

In a wok or large skillet, heat the oil over medium-high heat, swirling to coat the bottom. Cook the garlic and serrano pepper for 10 to 15 seconds, stirring constantly. Watch carefully so they don't burn.

Stir in the chicken. Cook for 3 to 4 minutes, or until the chicken is no longer pink in the center, stirring constantly.

Stir in the broccoli, carrots, and green onions. Cook for 2 to 3 minutes, or until the vegetables are tender-crisp, stirring constantly.

Stir in the reserved sauce and basil. Cook for 1 minute, or until the mixture is heated through, stirring constantly.

Serve the stir-fry over the rice.

COOK'S TIP ON THAI BASIL: Thai basil has a thin green leaf with a purplish cast. Look for it in Asian markets or specialty grocery stores, as well as at your local farmers' market. If it's not available, you can substitute sweet Italian basil, but the flavor will be different.

COOK'S TIP ON FISH SAUCE: Made from fermented fish soaked in brine, this sauce can best be described as having a pungent and saline taste. It imparts a rich flavor to many Asian dishes. Fortunately, given that it's extremely high in sodium, a little goes a very long way. Try to purchase a small bottle if you can. Store fish sauce in a cool place for up to six months.

PER SERVING

Calories 365	Cholesterol 73 mg	DIETARY EXCHANGES:
Total Fat 6.0 g	Sodium 454 mg	2½ starch
Saturated Fat 1.0 g	Carbohydrates 47 g	2 vegetable
Trans Fat 0.0 g	Fiber 6 g	3 lean meat
Polyunsaturated Fat 1.5 g	Sugars 6 g	
Monounsaturated Fat 2.0 g	Protein 30 g	

Greek-Style Stewed Chicken

Serves 4

Stock your kitchen with the flavors of Greece—tomatoes, olives, lemons, oregano—and you'll be ready to prepare this robust dish at any time. Serve with steamed green beans and whole-grain pita bread. While this dish is stewing to perfection, put together a healthy version of a classic Greek dessert, Mock Baklava (page 306), to finish off your meal.

- 1 teaspoon olive oil
- 1 pound chicken breast tenders, all visible fat discarded
- 1 medium green bell pepper, cut into 1-inch strips
- 2 medium shallots, quartered
- 1 14.5-ounce can no-salt-added diced tomatoes, undrained
- ½ cup fat-free, low-sodium chicken broth
- ¼ cup kalamata olives, coarsely chopped
- 1 teaspoon grated lemon zest
- 2 tablespoons fresh lemon juice
- 1 teaspoon dried oregano, crumbled
- ¼ teaspoon pepper
- ⅛ teaspoon salt
- ⅛ teaspoon ground cinnamon

In a large nonstick skillet, heat the oil over medium-high heat, swirling to coat the bottom. Cook the chicken for 2 minutes on each side.

Stir in the bell pepper and shallots. Cook for 2 to 3 minutes, or until the vegetables are tender-crisp, stirring occasionally.

Stir in the remaining ingredients, including the tomatoes with liquid. Bring to a simmer. Reduce the heat and simmer, covered, for 25 to 30 minutes, or until the chicken is no longer pink in the center.

PER SERVING

Calories 206	Cholesterol 73 mg	DIETARY EXCHANGES:
Total Fat 7.0 g	Sodium 428 mg	2 vegetable
Saturated Fat 1.0 g	Carbohydrates 10 g	3 lean meat
Trans Fat 0.0 g	Fiber 3 g	
Polyunsaturated Fat 1.0 g	Sugars 4 g	
Monounsaturated Fat 4.0 g	Protein 26 g	

Chicken and Veggie Bake

Serves 6

If you love chicken salad, you're sure to fall for this baked version. The hot, creamy sauce blankets bites of chicken and veggies as well as water chestnuts, which give the dish a pleasant crunch.

Cooking spray
2 tablespoons light tub margarine
8 ounces button mushrooms, sliced
½ cup diced green bell pepper
½ cup diced red bell pepper
½ cup chopped onion
½ cup slivered water chestnuts, drained
¼ cup whole-wheat panko (Japanese-style bread crumbs)
1 tablespoon shredded or grated Parmesan cheese
¼ cup light mayonnaise
2 teaspoons fresh lemon juice
½ teaspoon dried thyme, crumbled
Dash of pepper (white preferred)
2 cups diced cooked skinless chicken breast, cooked without salt, all visible fat discarded

Preheat the oven to 375°F. Lightly spray an 8-inch square baking dish with cooking spray.

In a nonstick skillet, melt the margarine over medium-high heat, swirling to coat the bottom. Cook the mushrooms, green and red bell pepper, onion, and water chestnuts, covered, for 7 to 9 minutes, stirring occasionally. Uncover and cook for 2 minutes, or until the liquid evaporates, stirring occasionally. Set aside.

In a small bowl, stir together the panko and Parmesan.

In a large bowl, stir together the mayonnaise, lemon juice, thyme, and pepper. Stir in the chicken and the mushroom mixture until well combined. Spoon into the baking dish. Sprinkle the panko mixture over all.

Bake for 20 minutes.

PER SERVING		
Calories 157	Cholesterol 44 mg	DIETARY EXCHANGES:
Total Fat 6.0 g	Sodium 174 mg	1 vegetable
Saturated Fat 1.0 g	Carbohydrates 9 g	2 lean meat
Trans Fat 0.0 g	Fiber 2 g	
Polyunsaturated Fat 2.5 g	Sugars 2 g	
Monounsaturated Fat 2.0 g	Protein 17 g	

Chicken and Vegetable Lasagna

Serves 6

Creamy, cheesy, and packed with unexpected bites of tender chicken and carrots, zucchini, and spinach, this lasagna-with-a-twist is sure to satisfy even the heartiest appetite. Using oven-ready noodles lets you skip a step.

Cooking spray
1 tablespoon olive oil
1 cup chopped onion
1 cup thinly sliced carrots
1 medium zucchini, thinly sliced
2 medium garlic cloves, minced
10 ounces frozen chopped spinach, thawed and squeezed dry
12 ounces cooked skinless chicken breast, cooked without salt, all visible fat discarded, shredded into bite-size pieces
⅓ cup all-purpose flour
¼ teaspoon pepper
15 ounces canned fat-free evaporated milk
2 cups fat-free, low-sodium chicken broth
¼ teaspoon salt
⅛ teaspoon ground nutmeg
¼ cup chopped fresh parsley
1 cup fat-free ricotta cheese
½ cup grated low-fat mozzarella cheese
9 oven-ready whole-grain lasagna noodles
½ cup shredded or grated Parmesan cheese

Preheat the oven to 350°F. Lightly spray a 9-inch square baking dish and a sheet of aluminum foil large enough to cover it with cooking spray. Set aside.

In a large nonstick skillet, heat the oil over medium heat, swirling to coat the bottom. Cook the onion and carrots for 6 minutes, or until softened, stirring frequently.

Stir in the zucchini and garlic. Cook for 3 minutes, or until the zucchini is tender, stirring frequently.

Stir in the spinach. Cook for 1 minute, using the back of a spoon to break up the clumps of spinach. Remove from the heat.

Stir in the chicken. Set aside.

Meanwhile, in a medium saucepan, stir together the flour and pepper. Slowly pour in the milk, whisking constantly. Add the broth, salt, and nutmeg, whisking until the mixture is smooth. Bring to a boil over medium-high heat, whisking constantly. Boil for 1 minute, or until slightly thickened, whisking constantly. Remove from the heat. Stir in the parsley.

In a small bowl, stir together the ricotta and mozzarella.

Spread 1 cup sauce in the dish. Arrange 3 lasagna noodles over the sauce (you may have to break one noodle in half lengthwise to fit). Spoon ⅓ cup sauce over the noodles, spreading evenly. Dot with one-third of the ricotta mixture, then one-third of the chicken mixture. Repeat the layers twice. Spread the remaining sauce over the top. Sprinkle with the Parmesan. Cover the baking dish with the aluminum foil with the sprayed side down.

Bake for 40 minutes. Remove the foil. Bake for 10 minutes, or until the Parmesan is lightly browned. Let stand for 10 minutes before serving.

....

COOK'S TIP: Don't worry if the sauce seems too runny. The oven-ready noodles need that extra moisture and will absorb it while the lasagna is baking.

....

PER SERVING

Calories 424	Cholesterol 60 mg	DIETARY EXCHANGES:
Total Fat 8.5 g	Sodium 541 mg	2 starch
Saturated Fat 2.5 g	Carbohydrates 45 g	½ fat-free milk
Trans Fat 0.0 g	Fiber 4 g	2 vegetable
Polyunsaturated Fat 1.0 g	Sugars 14 g	4 lean meat
Monounsaturated Fat 3.5 g	Protein 40 g	

Chicken Pot Pie with
Mashed Potato Topping

This pot pie trades the traditional pastry crust for a blanket of fluffy mashed potatoes seasoned with rosemary and nutmeg. It's a creative and delicious way to use up leftover cooked chicken breast and baked potatoes.

Cooking spray

½ **cup fat-free milk**

⅓ **cup all-purpose flour**

1 **cup water**

½ **teaspoon dried tarragon, crumbled**

½ **teaspoon dried parsley, crumbled**

½ **teaspoon pepper (freshly ground preferred)**

2 **cups diced cooked skinless chicken breast, cooked without salt, all visible fat discarded**

1 **16-ounce package of frozen mixed vegetables, such as carrots, lima beans, and peas, cooked using the package directions, omitting the salt**

¾ **cup cooked pearl onions**

TOPPING

2 **cups chopped cooked potatoes (russets preferred), cooked without salt**

½ **cup fat-free milk**

2 **tablespoons light tub margarine**

¼ **teaspoon pepper (freshly ground preferred)**

⅛ **teaspoon dried rosemary, crushed**

⅛ **teaspoon ground nutmeg**

⅛ **teaspoon paprika**

Preheat the oven to 400°F. Lightly spray a 1½-quart casserole dish with cooking spray.

In a saucepan, whisk together the milk and flour. Pour in the water, whisking to combine.

Stir in the tarragon, parsley, and pepper. Cook over medium heat for 3 to 5 minutes, or until thickened, stirring occasionally. Remove from the heat.

Stir in the chicken, mixed vegetables, and onions. Pour the mixture into the casserole dish.

In a large bowl, using an electric mixer on medium speed, beat together the topping ingredients except the paprika until light and fluffy. Spread the potato mixture over the chicken mixture. Sprinkle the paprika over all.

Bake for 20 minutes, or until the topping is lightly browned.

PER SERVING

Calories 359	Cholesterol 61 mg	DIETARY EXCHANGES:
Total Fat 5.5 g	Sodium 158 mg	2 starch
Saturated Fat 1.0 g	Carbohydrates 48 g	1 vegetable
Trans Fat 0.0 g	Fiber 6 g	3 lean meat
Polyunsaturated Fat 1.5 g	Sugars 9 g	
Monounsaturated Fat 2.0 g	Protein 30 g	

Cumin-Roasted Turkey Breast with Raspberry Sauce

Serves 6 (with half the turkey [about 18 ounces]
reserved for another use)

Frozen raspberries, available year-round, are the base for the lusciously fruity sauce that complements this perfectly seasoned entrée. Use the leftover turkey in whole-grain pita pockets, or substitute it for the chicken in Chicken Pot Pie with Mashed Potato Topping (page 172) or Chicken and Vegetable Lasagna (page 170).

Cooking spray
2 **teaspoons ground cumin**
½ **teaspoon garlic powder**
½ **teaspoon pepper**
¼ **teaspoon salt**
1 **4½-pound bone-in turkey breast with skin, thawed and patted dry with paper towels if frozen**

SAUCE

12 **ounces frozen unsweetened raspberries, thawed**
2 **teaspoons grated orange zest**
½ **cup fresh orange juice**
¼ **cup sugar**
2 **tablespoons balsamic vinegar**
1½ **tablespoons cornstarch**
¼ **teaspoon crushed red pepper flakes (optional)**
⅛ **teaspoon ground allspice**

Preheat the oven to 325°F. Lightly spray a large roasting pan with cooking spray (no rack needed).

In a small bowl, stir together the cumin, garlic powder, pepper, and salt.

Using your fingers, gently loosen but don't remove the turkey skin. Being careful to avoid tearing the skin, spread the cumin mixture over as much of the meat as possible. Gently pull the skin over any exposed meat. Put the turkey with the skin side up in the roasting pan.

Roast for 1 hour 25 minutes, or until the turkey registers 165°F on an instant-read thermometer and the juices run clear. For easier carving, let stand on a cooling rack for 15 minutes. Discard the skin. Cut the breast in half, thinly slicing one of the pieces and reserving the remaining piece for a later use.

Meanwhile, in a medium saucepan, stir together the sauce ingredients until the cornstarch is completely dissolved. Bring to a boil over medium-high heat. Boil for 1 minute, stirring frequently. Remove from the heat. Let cool completely.

Serve the turkey slices with the sauce.

. . . .

COOK'S TIP: If the turkey tips over when you put it in the baking dish, crumple a sheet of aluminum foil and wedge it under the turkey to stabilize it. A ball of foil placed in the cavity will work as well.

. . . .

PER SERVING

Calories 225	Cholesterol 80 mg	DIETARY EXCHANGES:
Total Fat 1.5 g	Sodium 152 mg	1 fruit
Saturated Fat 0.5 g	Carbohydrates 24 g	½ other carbohydrate
Trans Fat 0.0 g	Fiber 3 g	4 lean meat
Polyunsaturated Fat 0.5 g	Sugars 16 g	
Monounsaturated Fat 0.0 g	Protein 29 g	

Turkey Meatballs in Squash Shells

Serves 4

This dish features a white caper sauce and a slightly tart flavor. The meatballs are usually served with boiled potatoes and sometimes with beets, but this version is served in acorn squash halves. For a more traditional take, skip the squash and serve the meatballs with Beets in Orange Sauce (page 248).

2 small acorn squashes (about 1 pound each), halved, seeds and strings discarded

2 tablespoons water and ½ cup water, divided use

1 pound ground skinless turkey or chicken breast

1 cup plain soft whole-grain bread crumbs (about 2 slices of bread) (lowest sodium available)

¼ cup finely chopped onion

1 large egg

½ teaspoon Worcestershire sauce (lowest sodium available)

⅛ teaspoon salt

⅛ teaspoon pepper

1½ cups dry white wine (regular or nonalcoholic)

4 black peppercorns

3 whole cloves

1 medium dried bay leaf

Fat-free, low-sodium chicken broth or water (up to 1 cup)

2 tablespoons all-purpose flour

2 teaspoons capers, drained

Chopped fresh parsley

Place the squashes with the cut sides down in a microwaveable baking dish. Pierce the skins several times with a fork. Add 2 tablespoons water to the dish.

Microwave on 100 percent power (high) for 15 to 20 minutes, or until the squash can easily be pierced with the tip of a sharp knife, turning the dish twice during the cooking time. Drain.

Preheat the oven to 350°F.

Return the squash halves to the baking dish with the cut sides down. Bake for 30 minutes. Turn the cut sides up. Bake for 20 minutes, or until tender. Remove from the oven. Cover to keep warm. Set aside.

Meanwhile, crumble the turkey into a medium bowl. Add the bread crumbs, onion, egg, Worcestershire sauce, salt, and pepper. Using your hands or a spoon, combine the ingredients. Don't overwork the mixture or it will become too compact and the meatballs will be heavy. Shape into 24 meatballs. Transfer to a plate.

In a large skillet, stir together the wine, peppercorns, cloves, bay leaf, and the remaining ½ cup water. Bring to a boil over high heat. Reduce the heat to low. Add the meatballs and simmer, covered, for 10 minutes, or until the meatballs register 165°F on an instant-read thermometer. Transfer them to a separate plate. Cover to keep warm. Set aside.

Strain the liquid from the skillet into a measuring cup. Pour in enough broth to equal 1 cup.

Put the flour in a small bowl. Add ¼ cup of the liquid, whisking until smooth. Return the remaining liquid and the flour mixture to the skillet, whisking to blend. Cook over medium heat for 5 minutes, or until thickened and bubbly, whisking frequently.

Stir in the capers. Cook for 1 minute, stirring constantly. Return the meatballs to the skillet, spooning the sauce over them. Reduce the heat to low and cook for 2 minutes, or until the meatballs are heated through. Discard the peppercorns, cloves, and bay leaf.

Spoon the meatballs and sauce into the squash halves. Sprinkle with the parsley.

PER SERVING

Calories 281	Cholesterol 92 mg	DIETARY EXCHANGES:
Total Fat 3.5 g	Sodium 258 mg	2 starch
Saturated Fat 0.5 g	Carbohydrates 28 g	3 lean meat
Trans Fat 0.0 g	Fiber 4 g	
Polyunsaturated Fat 1.0 g	Sugars 5 g	
Monounsaturated Fat 1.0 g	Protein 33 g	

Turkey Patties with Fresh Basil-Mushroom Sauce

Serves 4

Thinly spread with Dijon mustard and containing a light sprinkle of chopped fresh basil, these turkey patties will surprise you with their layers of flavor. Serve a salad of dark, leafy greens with a cooling Creamy Herb Dressing (page 98) to complement the bit of heat in the slightly kicked-up mushroom sauce.

> 1 pound ground skinless turkey breast
> ¼ cup chopped fresh basil and 1 tablespoon chopped fresh basil, divided use
> ¼ teaspoon salt and ¼ teaspoon salt, divided use
> ¼ teaspoon garlic powder
> 1 tablespoon olive oil and 1½ teaspoons olive oil, divided use
> 8 ounces button mushrooms, sliced
> 1 large onion, chopped
> ⅛ teaspoon cayenne
> 2 teaspoons Dijon mustard (lowest sodium available)

Crumble the turkey into a medium bowl. Add ¼ cup basil, ¼ teaspoon salt, and the garlic powder. Using your hands or a spoon, combine the ingredients. Shape into 4 patties.

In a large nonstick skillet, heat 1 tablespoon oil over medium-high heat, swirling to coat the bottom. Cook the patties for 5 minutes. Turn over the patties. Cook for 4 minutes, or until the patties register 165°F on an instant-read thermometer. Transfer to a plate. Cover to keep warm.

In the same skillet, still over medium-high heat, heat the remaining 1½ teaspoons oil, swirling to coat the bottom. Cook the mushrooms, onion, and cayenne for 4 minutes, or until the onion is soft, stirring frequently. Remove from the heat. Stir in the remaining 1 tablespoon basil and ¼ teaspoon salt. Just before serving, spread the mustard over the patties. Top with the mushroom mixture.

PER SERVING

Calories 208	Cholesterol 77 mg	DIETARY EXCHANGES:
Total Fat 6.5 g	Sodium 397 mg	1 vegetable
Saturated Fat 1.0 g	Carbohydrates 7 g	3 lean meat
Trans Fat 0.0 g	Fiber 2 g	
Polyunsaturated Fat 1.0 g	Sugars 4 g	
Monounsaturated Fat 4.0 g	Protein 30 g	

Meats

BEEF TENDERLOIN ROAST 180

GRILLED TERIYAKI SIRLOIN 182

GRILLED SIRLOIN STEAK WITH CHIMICHURRI SAUCE 184

SPICED SHISH KEBABS WITH HORSERADISH CREAM 186

BALSAMIC BRAISED BEEF WITH EXOTIC MUSHROOMS 188

SIRLOIN STEAK WITH PORTOBELLO MUSHROOMS 189

SLOW-COOKER PEPPER STEAK 190

BULGUR AND GROUND BEEF CASSEROLE 191

MEAT LOAF WITH APRICOT GLAZE 192

STUFFED CABBAGE ROLLS 194

MEATBALLS HAWAIIAN 196

SOUTHWESTERN BEEF PITA TACOS 198

CHILI 200

BUNLESS BEEF-AND-BEAN BURGERS 202

PORK WITH SAVORY SAUCE 203

HAM AND RICE CROQUETTES 204

PORK WITH CORN-CILANTRO PESTO 206

SPICY BAKED PORK CHOPS 208

SKILLET PORK CHOPS WITH CINNAMON-APPLE SALSA 209

PORK AND PEPPER STEW 210

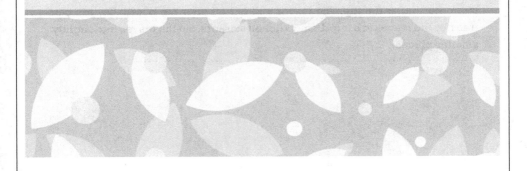

Beef Tenderloin Roast

Serves 8

Enhanced by a tangy and slightly spicy rub, this beef roast is ideal for holidays or just dinner at home with the family. Try it with Roasted Brussels Sprouts (page 252) and Sweet Potatoes in Creamy Cinnamon Sauce (page 263), which can cook alongside the beef. Cherry-Pear Turnovers (page 300) are a lusciously fruity final course.

Cooking spray

RUB

¼ cup chopped fresh rosemary

¼ cup Dijon mustard (lowest sodium available)

¼ cup bottled white horseradish, drained

2 tablespoons pink peppercorns, crushed, or 2 teaspoons black pepper (coarsely ground preferred)

1 tablespoon onion powder

4 medium garlic cloves, minced

2 teaspoons olive oil

. . . .

1 2-pound beef tenderloin, all visible fat and silver skin discarded

Preheat the oven to 400°F. Lightly spray a heavy roasting pan with cooking spray (no rack needed).

In a small bowl, stir together the rub ingredients. Coat the beef with the rub. Transfer to the roasting pan.

Roast for 40 minutes to 1 hour 5 minutes, or to the desired doneness. Transfer the beef to a cutting board. Let stand for 10 minutes before cutting the beef crosswise into thin slices.

COOK'S TIP ON FRESH ROSEMARY: To chop fresh rosemary, hold a thick, woody stem upright over your cutting board at a slight angle so the leaves are pointing upward. Run your index finger and thumb down the length of the stem, starting at the top. The leaves will fall off onto the board. Or, you can transfer the leaves to a cup. Using kitchen scissors, cut the leaves into slightly smaller pieces.

COOK'S TIP ON PEPPERCORNS: Peppercorns are actually berries produced on the vines of pepper plants. Depending on when they're picked, the berries vary quite a bit in flavor. The green peppercorn is mild and fresh tasting. The common black peppercorn is pungent, yet slightly sweet. For a mild-flavored pepper, try the white peppercorn. Pink peppercorns add a flavorful touch (similar to that of black pepper) to sauces and other dishes. They aren't true peppercorns; they're the dried berries from a rose-family plant traditionally cultivated in Madagascar.

PER SERVING

Calories 173	Cholesterol 59 mg	DIETARY EXCHANGES:
Total Fat 7.5 g	Sodium 229 mg	3 lean meat
Saturated Fat 2.5 g	Carbohydrates 4 g	
Trans Fat 0.0 g	Fiber 1 g	
Polyunsaturated Fat 0.5 g	Sugars 1 g	
Monounsaturated Fat 3.0 g	Protein 22 g	

Grilled Teriyaki Sirloin

Fire up the grill for this Japanese-inspired steak, which is topped with nutty sesame seeds and accompanied by plump sugar snap peas tossed with toasted sesame oil. Serve with brown rice, or grill some extra vegetables alongside the beef.

MARINADE

- 2 tablespoons soy sauce (lowest sodium available)
- 1 tablespoon dry sherry or white wine vinegar
- 2 medium garlic cloves, minced
- 1 teaspoon grated peeled gingerroot or ¼ teaspoon ground ginger
- 1 teaspoon light brown sugar
- 1 teaspoon toasted sesame oil
  ....
- 4 boneless sirloin steaks (about 4 ounces each), all visible fat discarded
  Cooking spray
- 6 ounces sugar snap peas, trimmed
- ¼ cup water
- ½ teaspoon toasted sesame oil
- 1 tablespoon sesame seeds, dry-roasted

In a shallow glass dish, whisk together the marinade ingredients. Add the beef, turning to coat. Cover and refrigerate for 15 minutes to 8 hours, turning occasionally.

When the beef has marinated, lightly spray the grill rack with cooking spray. Preheat the grill on medium high.

Drain the beef, discarding the marinade. Grill the beef for 4 to 7 minutes on each side, or until the desired doneness. Transfer to a cutting board. Cover to keep warm.

In a medium microwaveable bowl, microwave the peas and water, covered, on 100 percent power (high) for 1 minute, or until the peas are tender-crisp. Drain well in a colander. Return the peas to the bowl. Stir in the sesame oil.

Serve the beef with the peas. Sprinkle with the sesame seeds.

....

COOK'S TIP ON GINGERROOT: If the produce section of your grocery store has only large pieces of gingerroot, it's appropriate to break off what you need. Use a spoon, knife, or vegetable peeler to remove the skin before grating the flesh.

....

PER SERVING

Calories 170	Cholesterol 56 mg	DIETARY EXCHANGES:
Total Fat 6.0 g	Sodium 245 mg	1 vegetable
Saturated Fat 2.0 g	Carbohydrates 5 g	3 lean meat
Trans Fat 0.0 g	Fiber 1 g	
Polyunsaturated Fat 1.0 g	Sugars 3 g	
Monounsaturated Fat 2.5 g	Protein 23 g	

Grilled Sirloin Steak with Chimichurri Sauce

Serves 4

In Argentina, chimichurri is commonly used both as a marinade and as a sauce to accompany grilled meats. It's usually made with fresh parsley, garlic, olive oil, and a touch of vinegar, but this version sweetens the pot with orange juice and a hint of brown sugar that perfectly complements seasoned sirloin steak.

SAUCE

- 1 cup loosely packed fresh parsley
- 2 tablespoons red wine vinegar
- 2 tablespoons fresh orange juice
- 1 teaspoon light brown sugar
- 1 teaspoon olive oil
- 1 medium garlic clove

. . . .

Cooking spray
- 1 teaspoon dried thyme, crumbled
- 1 teaspoon dried oregano, crumbled
- ½ teaspoon pepper
- ¼ teaspoon salt
- 4 boneless sirloin steaks (about 4 ounces each), all visible fat discarded

In a food processor or blender, process the sauce ingredients for 20 to 30 seconds, or until the parsley is finely chopped. Pour the mixture into an airtight container and refrigerate until serving time.

Lightly spray the grill rack with cooking spray. Preheat the grill on medium high.

Meanwhile, in a small bowl, stir together the thyme, oregano, pepper, and salt. Sprinkle over both sides of the beef. Using your fingertips, gently press the mixture so it adheres to the beef.

Grill the beef for 3 to 5 minutes on each side, or until the desired doneness. Serve with the sauce.

COOK'S TIP ON HEALTHY CUTS OF STEAK: Steak on a cholesterol-lowering diet? Sure. Just select lean cuts of meat, trim away all the visible fat, and limit your consumption. Besides sirloin steak, tenderloin, eye-of-round, and round steak are wise choices.

PER SERVING

Calories 152
Total Fat 5.0 g
  Saturated Fat 1.5 g
  Trans Fat 0.0 g
  Polyunsaturated Fat 0.5 g
  Monounsaturated Fat 2.5 g

Cholesterol 56 mg
Sodium 198 mg
Carbohydrates 4 g
  Fiber 1 g
  Sugars 2 g
Protein 22 g

DIETARY EXCHANGES:
3 lean meat

Spiced Shish Kebabs with Horseradish Cream

Serves 4

These spicy kebabs get their heat from a liberal dose of chili powder and the accompanying horseradish-spiked sauce. Cool things off by serving Very Berry Sorbet (page 317) or Strawberry Margarita Ice (page 318) for dessert.

HORSERADISH CREAM

⅓ cup fat-free sour cream
2 tablespoons light mayonnaise
1 tablespoon bottled white horseradish, drained
½ teaspoon garlic powder
Chili powder to taste
. . . .
1 pound boneless top sirloin steak, all visible fat discarded, cut into 16 cubes
2 teaspoons dried oregano, crumbled
1 teaspoon ground cumin
2 teaspoons chili powder
¾ teaspoon garlic powder
Cooking spray
½ large red onion, cut into 16 1-inch squares
1 large yellow bell pepper, cut into 16 1-inch squares
16 cherry or grape tomatoes

In a small serving bowl, whisk together the horseradish cream ingredients except the chili powder. Sprinkle with the chili powder. Cover and refrigerate until serving time.

Put the beef in a shallow casserole dish. In a small bowl, stir together the oregano, cumin, and the remaining 2 teaspoons chili powder and ¾ teaspoon garlic powder. Sprinkle the mixture all over the beef. Using your fingertips, gently press the mixture so it adheres to the beef. Cover and refrigerate for 15 minutes.

Meanwhile, soak four 10- to 12-inch wooden skewers for at least 10 minutes in cold water to keep them from charring, or use metal skewers.

Preheat the broiler. Lightly spray the broiler pan and rack with cooking spray.

Thread each skewer with 4 beef cubes, 4 onion squares, 4 bell pepper squares, and 4 tomatoes, alternating the ingredients. Transfer the kebabs to the broiler rack.

Broil about 4 inches from the heat for 4 minutes. Turn over the kebabs. Broil for 3 minutes, or until the desired doneness. Serve with the horseradish cream.

PER SERVING

Calories 206	Cholesterol 62 mg	DIETARY EXCHANGES:
Total Fat 6.5 g	Sodium 172 mg	½ starch
Saturated Fat 1.5 g	Carbohydrates 13 g	1 vegetable
Trans Fat 0.0 g	Fiber 2 g	3 lean meat
Polyunsaturated Fat 1.5 g	Sugars 5 g	
Monounsaturated Fat 2.0 g	Protein 24 g	

Balsamic Braised Beef with Exotic Mushrooms

Serves 4

Slow, gentle braising makes the lean meat in this recipe fork-tender, while the braising liquid becomes a savory sauce. Try it on a bed of whole-grain pasta, brown rice, or farro.

1 1-pound boneless eye-of-round or sirloin steak, all visible fat discarded

1 pound mixed mushrooms, such as enoki, oyster, portobello, shiitake (stems discarded), wood ear, and button, larger mushrooms cut into ¼-inch slices

1 cup fat-free, low-sodium beef broth

2 tablespoons balsamic vinegar

1 tablespoon chopped fresh rosemary or 1 teaspoon dried rosemary, crushed

1 teaspoon onion powder

1 teaspoon garlic powder

1 medium dried bay leaf

2 tablespoons all-purpose flour

¼ cup water

In a large nonstick skillet, cook the beef over medium-high heat for 2 minutes on each side.

Stir in the mushrooms. Cook for 2 to 3 minutes, or until the mushrooms are slightly soft, stirring occasionally. Stir in the broth, vinegar, rosemary, onion powder, garlic powder, and bay leaf. Bring to a simmer, stirring occasionally. Reduce the heat and simmer, covered, for 45 to 50 minutes, or until the beef is tender.

Put the flour in a small bowl. Add the water, whisking until smooth. Pour into the beef mixture. Increase the heat to medium high and cook for 2 to 3 minutes, or until the sauce is thickened, stirring occasionally. Discard the bay leaf.

PER SERVING

Calories 198	Cholesterol 66 mg	DIETARY EXCHANGES:
Total Fat 4.0 g	Sodium 73 mg	2 vegetable
Saturated Fat 1.5 g	Carbohydrates 10 g	3 lean meat
Trans Fat 0.0 g	Fiber 2 g	
Polyunsaturated Fat 0.5 g	Sugars 4 g	
Monounsaturated Fat 1.5 g	Protein 31 g	

Sirloin Steak with Portobello Mushrooms

Serves 4

Peppery sirloin is cooked to perfection, then smothered in meaty portobellos and sweet onions bathed in a rich, zesty sauce. Pair this with low-fat mashed potatoes or a whole grain such as bulgur to soak up every drop of the sauce. Be sure to round out the meal with a no-fuss vegetable, such as Wilted Spinach (page 268) or Apple-Lemon Carrots (page 255).

1 teaspoon dried thyme, crumbled

½ teaspoon pepper (coarsely ground preferred)

4 boneless sirloin steaks (about 4 ounces each), all visible fat discarded

8 ounces portobello mushrooms, cut into 1-inch squares

1 large red onion, sliced

½ cup fat-free, low-sodium beef broth

2 tablespoons brandy (optional)

1 tablespoon Dijon mustard (lowest sodium available)

1 tablespoon Worcestershire sauce (lowest sodium available)

Sprinkle the thyme and pepper over both sides of the beef.

Heat a large nonstick skillet over medium-high heat. Cook the beef for 4 to 6 minutes on each side, or to the desired doneness. Transfer to a platter. Cover to keep warm.

In the same skillet, still over medium-high heat, cook the mushrooms and onion for 1 to 2 minutes, or until the onion is almost soft, stirring occasionally.

Stir in the remaining ingredients. Cook for 5 to 6 minutes, or until the mushrooms are soft and the liquid is reduced by half (to about ⅜ cup), stirring occasionally. Spoon over the beef.

PER SERVING

Calories 164	Cholesterol 56 mg	DIETARY EXCHANGES:
Total Fat 4.5 g	Sodium 159 mg	1 vegetable
Saturated Fat 1.5 g	Carbohydrates 8 g	3 lean meat
Trans Fat 0.0 g	Fiber 2 g	
Polyunsaturated Fat 0.0 g	Sugars 4 g	
Monounsaturated Fat 1.5 g	Protein 23 g	

Slow-Cooker Pepper Steak

Serves 4

Cherry tomatoes stirred in just before serving add a burst of freshness to this Asian-style one-dish meal. If you'd like, start your meal with Hot-and-Sour Soup with Exotic Mushrooms (page 64).

- 1 pound boneless top round steak, all visible fat discarded, cut into thin strips
- 2 cups fat-free, low-sodium beef broth
- 1 medium red bell pepper, cut into 1-inch strips
- 1 medium green bell pepper, cut into 1-inch strips
- ½ medium onion, cut into 1-inch strips
- 2 tablespoons soy sauce (lowest sodium available)
- 1 teaspoon toasted sesame oil
- ¼ teaspoon crushed red pepper flakes (optional)
- 1 cup uncooked instant brown rice
- 1 cup cherry tomatoes, whole or halved

In a 3½- to 4-quart round or oval slow cooker, stir together the beef, broth, bell peppers, onion, soy sauce, sesame oil, and red pepper flakes. Cook, covered, on low for 6 to 8 hours or on high for 2 to 3 hours.

If using the low setting, change it to high. Quickly stir in the rice. Cook for 5 minutes, or until the rice is tender.

Just before serving, stir in the cherry tomatoes.

. . . .

COOK'S TIP: To halve or not to halve—that is the question when cooking with cherry tomatoes. If left whole, they provide more intense flavor when you bite into them. If halved, they tend to soak up flavors from sauces, dressings, and marinades.

. . . .

PER SERVING

Calories 263	Cholesterol 57 mg	DIETARY EXCHANGES:
Total Fat 5.5 g	Sodium 296 mg	1 starch
Saturated Fat 1.5 g	Carbohydrates 25 g	2 vegetable
Trans Fat 0.0 g	Fiber 3 g	3 lean meat
Polyunsaturated Fat 1.0 g	Sugars 6 g	
Monounsaturated Fat 2.0 g	Protein 28 g	

Bulgur and Ground Beef Casserole

Serves 4

A whole grain beefs up this meaty casserole, providing a nutty flavor and filling fiber. Pair it with Cauliflower au Gratin (page 256) or your favorite steamed vegetable.

Cooking spray
1 pound extra-lean ground beef
2 medium onions, chopped
4 medium tomatoes, chopped
1 cup uncooked instant, or fine-grain, bulgur
½ cup finely chopped fresh cilantro or parsley
½ cup low-sodium mixed-vegetable juice
2 tablespoons fresh lemon juice
1 tablespoon chopped fresh dillweed or 1 heaping teaspoon dried dillweed, crumbled
¼ teaspoon salt
¼ teaspoon plus ⅛ teaspoon garlic powder
¼ teaspoon pepper

Preheat the oven to 350°F.

Lightly spray a Dutch oven with cooking spray. Cook the beef over medium-high heat for 4 to 5 minutes, or until the beef is browned on the outside and no longer pink in the center, stirring occasionally to turn and break up the beef.

Stir the onions into the beef. Cook for 3 to 4 minutes, or until the onions are soft, stirring occasionally. Remove from the heat.

Stir in the remaining ingredients. Spoon the beef mixture into a 9-inch square or 11 x 7 x 2-inch baking dish.

Bake for 15 to 20 minutes, or until heated through.

PER SERVING

Calories 322	Cholesterol 62 mg	DIETARY EXCHANGES:
Total Fat 6.5 g	Sodium 265 mg	2 starch
Saturated Fat 2.5 g	Carbohydrates 40 g	2 vegetable
Trans Fat 0.5 g	Fiber 10 g	3 lean meat
Polyunsaturated Fat 1.0 g	Sugars 9 g	
Monounsaturated Fat 2.5 g	Protein 31 g	

Meat Loaf with Apricot Glaze

Serves 6

A grated apple is the surprise ingredient that helps make this meat loaf extra moist. The spicy-sweet apricot glaze provides the finishing touch. Try this with Praline Butternut Squash (page 266) or Individual Corn Puddings (page 259), which bake at the same temperature, so you can have everything ready at the same time.

Cooking spray

MEAT LOAF

- 1 **pound extra-lean ground beef**
- ½ **cup uncooked quick-cooking oatmeal**
- 1 **small onion, grated (about ½ cup)**
- 1 **small apple, peeled and grated (about ½ cup)**
- 2 **large egg whites**
- 2 **tablespoons chopped fresh parsley**
- 2 **tablespoons Worcestershire sauce (lowest sodium available)**
- 2 **tablespoons no-salt-added ketchup**
- 2 **medium garlic cloves, minced**
- 1 **teaspoon dried oregano, crumbled**
- ¼ **teaspoon salt**

GLAZE

- ½ **cup all-fruit apricot spread**
- 3 **tablespoons no-salt-added ketchup**
- 2 **tablespoons fresh orange juice**
- 1 **tablespoon honey**
- 2 **teaspoons cornstarch**
- ½ **teaspoon ground ginger**
- ¼ **teaspoon red hot-pepper sauce**

Preheat the oven to 350°F. Lightly spray a 9 x 5 x 3-inch loaf pan with cooking spray.

Crumble the beef into a large bowl. Add the remaining meat loaf ingredients. Using your hands or a spoon, combine the ingredients.

Transfer the beef mixture to the pan. Lightly pat the meat loaf into a rectangle slightly smaller than the pan.

Bake for 45 minutes (the meat loaf won't be done at this point). Remove from the oven. Pour off and discard any fat.

Meanwhile, in a small saucepan, whisk together the glaze ingredients. Cook over medium-high heat for 8 to 10 minutes, or until thickened and bubbling, whisking constantly.

Spoon the glaze over the cooked meat loaf.

Bake for 15 minutes, or until the meat loaf reaches an internal temperature of 160°F on an instant-read thermometer. Remove from the oven. Let stand for 5 to 10 minutes before slicing.

COOK'S TIP: You can easily double this recipe and make two meat loaves. Cook both at the same time, then freeze the extra one to have on hand for a busy day.

PER SERVING

Calories 268	Cholesterol 43 mg	DIETARY EXCHANGES:
Total Fat 8.5 g	Sodium 200 mg	2 other carbohydrate
Saturated Fat 3.0 g	Carbohydrates 31 g	2½ lean meat
Trans Fat 0.0 g	Fiber 2 g	
Polyunsaturated Fat 0.5 g	Sugars 20 g	
Monounsaturated Fat 3.0 g	Protein 17 g	

Stuffed Cabbage Rolls

Serves 4

Some version of stuffed cabbage is common to many regions, including Eastern Europe, the Mediterranean, the Middle East, and even Asia. In this Greek rendition, crunchy pine nuts and plump raisins add texture and flavor to the beef-and-rice filling. While the cabbage rolls bake, make Zucchini Spread (page 36) to use up some of the extra fresh parsley.

  1 **cup uncooked brown rice**
  1 **medium head of green cabbage**
  ½ **pound extra-lean ground beef**
  1 **teaspoon olive oil and 1 teaspoon olive oil, divided use**
  1 **large onion, chopped**
  ¼ **cup plus 2 tablespoons dried mint, crumbled**
  3 **tablespoons fresh lemon juice**
  2 **tablespoons minced fresh parsley and 2 tablespoons minced fresh parsley, divided use**
1½ **tablespoons raisins**
  1 **tablespoon pine nuts**
  ½ **teaspoon ground cinnamon**
  ¼ **teaspoon pepper, or to taste**
  ⅛ **teaspoon salt**
  2 **cups marinara sauce (lowest sodium available)**

Prepare the rice using the package directions, omitting the salt and margarine. Fluff with a fork. Set aside.

Using a sharp paring knife, remove the core of the cabbage. Bring a large stockpot of water to a boil over high heat. Carefully add the cabbage, turning to ensure that the boiling water gets into the leaves around the core area. Boil for 10 minutes. Drain the cabbage well. Set aside to cool.

In a large skillet, cook the beef over medium heat for about 5 minutes, or until no longer pink, stirring occasionally to turn and break up the beef (the beef won't be done at this point). Transfer to a plate.

Wipe the skillet with paper towels. Heat 1 teaspoon oil over medium heat, swirling to coat the bottom. Cook the onion for 3 minutes, or until almost soft, stirring occasionally. Stir in the beef. Cook for about 2 minutes, or until the beef is browned, stirring occasionally. Stir in the mint, lemon juice, 2 tablespoons parsley, raisins, pine nuts, cinnamon, pepper, and salt. Add the cooked rice, stirring until well combined.

Preheat the oven to 350°F.

Pull 12 large leaves off the cabbage. Put 8 leaves on a flat surface with the stem end toward you. Gently cut out any large veins at the stem end of the leaves, then pull the sides together. Place a scant ½ cup of the beef mixture on each leaf toward the base. Fold the edges of the leaves toward the center so they slightly overlap. Trying to keep the cabbage rolls fairly tight, roll up from the stem end. Use a wooden toothpick to secure the roll if necessary.

Transfer the rolls with the seam side down to a 13 x 9 x 2-inch baking dish. Pour the marinara sauce over the rolls. Place the remaining 4 cabbage leaves over the rolls and sauce, tucking them in slightly on the sides to enclose the rolls and sauce. Brush the top of the leaves with the remaining 1 teaspoon oil. Bake for 1 hour.

Arrange the cabbage leaves covering the dish on a serving platter. Transfer the rolls and sauce to the platter. Sprinkle the remaining 2 tablespoons parsley over all.

PER SERVING

Calories 417	Cholesterol 38 mg	DIETARY EXCHANGES:
Total Fat 9.5 g	Sodium 264 mg	3 starch
Saturated Fat 2.5 g	Carbohydrates 65 g	4 vegetable
Trans Fat 0.5 g	Fiber 10 g	2 lean meat
Polyunsaturated Fat 2.0 g	Sugars 17 g	
Monounsaturated Fat 4.0 g	Protein 22 g	

Meatballs Hawaiian

Serves 6

Pineapple chunks add tropical flair to ginger-spiked meatballs simmered in a sweet soy-flavored sauce and ladled atop a bed of brown rice. Serve with Sweet-and-Sour Broccoli and Red Bell Pepper (page 251).

Cooking spray

MEATBALLS

- 1 **pound extra-lean ground beef**
- ½ **cup whole-wheat panko (Japanese-style bread crumbs)**
- 3 **tablespoons finely chopped green onions**
- 1¼ **teaspoons garlic powder**
- 1¼ **teaspoons grated peeled gingerroot**
  Pepper to taste
- 1 **large egg**

. . . .

- 1 **cup uncooked instant brown rice**
- 1 **8-ounce can pineapple chunks in their own juice, drained and juice reserved**
- ¼ **cup firmly packed brown sugar**
- 2 **tablespoons cornstarch**
- ¼ **cup white wine vinegar**
- 1 **teaspoon soy sauce (lowest sodium available)**
- 2 **medium green bell peppers, cut into thin strips or rings**

Preheat the broiler. Lightly spray the broiler pan and rack with cooking spray.

Crumble the beef into a medium bowl. Add the remaining meatball ingredients except the egg. Using your hands or a spoon, gently combine the ingredients. Don't overwork the mixture or it will become too compact and the meatballs will be heavy. Gently work in the egg. Shape into twelve ½-inch balls. Transfer to the broiler rack.

Broil the meatballs about 4 inches from the heat for about 15 minutes, or until the tops are browned. Turn over the meatballs. Broil for about 15 minutes, or until the meatballs are browned on the outside and no longer pink in the center. Drain on paper towels.

Meanwhile, prepare the rice using the package directions, omitting the salt and margarine. Set aside.

Put the reserved pineapple juice in a measuring cup. Add enough water to make 1 cup. Pour into a large nonstick skillet. Stir in the brown sugar, cornstarch, vinegar, and soy sauce. Cook over medium heat for 3 minutes, or until the sauce is thickened, stirring constantly. Stir in the pineapple, bell peppers, and cooked meatballs. Reduce the heat and simmer, covered, for 10 minutes.

Spoon the rice onto plates. Ladle the meatballs and sauce over the rice.

PER SERVING

Calories 267	Cholesterol 73 mg	DIETARY EXCHANGES:
Total Fat 5.0 g	Sodium 110 mg	1½ starch
Saturated Fat 2.0 g	Carbohydrates 35 g	1 other carbohydrate
Trans Fat 0.0 g	Fiber 2 g	2½ lean meat
Polyunsaturated Fat 1.0 g	Sugars 15 g	
Monounsaturated Fat 2.0 g	Protein 20 g	

Southwestern Beef Pita Tacos

Serves 6

Are they pita pockets or tacos? Either way, they're delicious! In this kid-friendly dish, we stuff whole-grain pita halves with taco-seasoned ground beef and fresh veggies. Serve with a side of Jícama and Grapefruit Salad with Ancho-Honey Dressing (page 80) and finish your meal with Strawberry Margarita Ice (page 318).

FILLING

    1 **pound extra-lean ground beef**
    1 **tablespoon all-purpose flour**
    1 **cup water**
    1 **teaspoon chili powder**
  ½ **teaspoon ground cumin**
  ¼ **teaspoon garlic powder**
  ¼ **teaspoon onion powder**
  ¼ **teaspoon pepper**
    . . . .
    6 **6-inch whole-grain pita pockets, halved**

TOPPINGS

 1½ **cups shredded romaine**
    2 **medium tomatoes, chopped (about 1 cup)**
  ½ **cup chopped green bell pepper**
  ½ **cup chopped onion**

Preheat the oven to 350°F.

In a large nonstick skillet, cook the beef over medium-high heat for 8 to 10 minutes, or until browned on the outside and no longer pink in the center, stirring occasionally to turn and break up the beef. Sprinkle with the flour, stirring to combine.

Stir in the remaining filling ingredients. Bring to a simmer, still over medium-high heat, stirring occasionally. Cook for 3 to 4 minutes, or until the mixture has thickened, stirring occasionally.

Meanwhile, wrap the pita halves in aluminum foil. Bake for 5 minutes, or until warm.

Spoon the filling into the pita halves. Sprinkle with the toppings.

PER SERVING

Calories 284
Total Fat 5.5 g
  Saturated Fat 2.0 g
  Trans Fat 0.0 g
  Polyunsaturated Fat 1.0 g
  Monounsaturated Fat 2.0 g

Cholesterol 42 mg
Sodium 389 mg
Carbohydrates 38 g
  Fiber 6 g
  Sugars 3 g
Protein 23 g

DIETARY EXCHANGES:
2 starch
1 vegetable
2½ lean meat

Chili

Every cook has a favorite chili recipe, but with its lean beef, beans, and just the right amount of smoky spice, this one will become yours. Like many other soups and stews, it tastes best when made in advance, allowing time for the flavors to blend. Serve with a side of Speckled Spoon Bread (page 280).

Cooking spray
1 pound extra-lean ground beef
2 large onions, chopped
2 8-ounce cans no-salt-added tomato sauce
1½ cups water and ¼ cup water, divided use
2 to 4 medium garlic cloves, minced
2 15.5-ounce cans no-salt-added pinto beans, rinsed and drained
3 tablespoons chili powder
1 or 2 medium fresh jalapeños, seeds and ribs discarded, chopped (optional; see Cook's Tip on page 101)
1 tablespoon chopped fresh oregano or 1 teaspoon dried oregano, crumbled
1 teaspoon ground cumin
½ teaspoon salt
⅛ teaspoon cayenne, or to taste
Pepper to taste
2 tablespoons cornstarch

Lightly spray a large, heavy saucepan or Dutch oven with cooking spray. Cook the beef over medium-high heat for 4 to 5 minutes, or until browned on the outside and no longer pink in the center, stirring occasionally to turn and break up the beef. Transfer the beef to a plate. Remove the pan from the heat.

Wipe the pan with paper towels. Lightly spray the pan with cooking spray. Return it to the heat.

Cook the onions, still over medium-high heat, for about 3 minutes, or until soft, stirring frequently.

Stir in the beef, tomato sauce, 1½ cups water, and the garlic. Reduce the heat and simmer, partially covered, for 20 minutes.

Stir in the beans, chili powder, jalapeño, oregano, cumin, salt, cayenne, and pepper. Simmer, partially covered, for 30 minutes.

Put the cornstarch in a small bowl. Add the remaining ¼ cup water, whisking to dissolve. Stir into the chili. Cook for 3 to 4 minutes, or until the chili is the desired consistency.

PER SERVING

Calories 298	Cholesterol 42 mg	DIETARY EXCHANGES:
Total Fat 4.5 g	Sodium 331 mg	2 starch
Saturated Fat 1.5 g	Carbohydrates 39 g	2 vegetable
Trans Fat 0.0 g	Fiber 10 g	3 lean meat
Polyunsaturated Fat 1.0 g	Sugars 12 g	
Monounsaturated Fat 1.5 g	Protein 27 g	

Bunless Beef-and-Bean Burgers

Serves 4

Using canned beans to replace some of the beef results in burgers with more fiber and less saturated fat. Their beefy flavor still comes through, so you won't miss the extra meat.

1　15.5-ounce can no-salt-added black beans or no-salt-added pinto beans, rinsed and drained

8　ounces extra-lean ground beef

¼　cup plain dry whole-grain bread crumbs (lowest sodium available)

2　teaspoons chili powder

1　teaspoon ground cumin

1　medium garlic clove, minced

¼　teaspoon salt

⅛　teaspoon pepper

2　teaspoons canola or corn oil

2　tablespoons chopped fresh cilantro

1　medium green onion, thinly sliced

1　medium fresh jalapeño, seeds and ribs discarded, minced (see Cook's Tip on page 101)

1　large tomato, cut crosswise into 4 thick slices

1　medium lime, cut into 4 wedges

In a medium bowl, using a potato masher or fork, mash the beans until slightly chunky. Add the beef, bread crumbs, chili powder, cumin, garlic, salt, and pepper. Using your hands or a spoon, combine the ingredients. Shape into 4 burgers, each about 4 inches in diameter.

In a large nonstick skillet, heat the oil over medium heat, swirling to coat the bottom. Cook the burgers, covered, for 4 to 5 minutes on each side, or until no longer pink in the center.

In a small bowl, stir together the cilantro, green onion, and jalapeño. Put the tomato slices on plates. Top the tomatoes with the burgers. Sprinkle the burgers with the cilantro mixture. Serve with the lime wedges.

PER SERVING

Calories 233	Cholesterol 31 mg	DIETARY EXCHANGES:
Total Fat 5.5 g	Sodium 221 mg	1½ starch
Saturated Fat 1.5 g	Carbohydrates 27 g	1 vegetable
Trans Fat 0.0 g	Fiber 7 g	2 lean meat
Polyunsaturated Fat 1.0 g	Sugars 7 g	
Monounsaturated Fat 2.5 g	Protein 20 g	

Pork with Savory Sauce

Serves 4

Wine and fruit-flavored vinegar combine to form a sauce that's just sweet enough to enhance the flavor of the pork without overpowering it. Carrot and Barley Pilaf (page 254) and Stir-Fried Cabbage with Noodles (page 253) are quick side dishes that can be prepared while the sauce is reducing.

- ¾ cup fat-free, low-sodium chicken broth
- ¼ cup raspberry or balsamic vinegar
- 2 tablespoons port wine or 100% grape juice
- 1 teaspoon olive oil
- ½ teaspoon pepper (coarsely ground preferred)
- ½ teaspoon dried oregano, crumbled
- 1 medium garlic clove, minced
- 1 teaspoon cornstarch
- 2 tablespoons water
- 1 pound pork tenderloin, all visible fat discarded, cut into ¼-inch-thick medallions

In a small saucepan, stir together the broth, vinegar, port, oil, pepper, oregano, and garlic. Cook over medium-high heat for 20 minutes, or until reduced by about half (to about ½ cup).

Put the cornstarch in a small bowl. Add the water, whisking to dissolve. Whisk into the sauce. Reduce the heat to medium. Cook for 1 minute, or until thickened, whisking constantly. Remove from the heat. Cover to keep warm.

Heat a large nonstick skillet over medium-high heat. Cook the pork for 3 to 4 minutes on each side, or until it registers 145°F on an instant-read thermometer. Remove from the heat. Let stand for 3 minutes. Serve with the sauce.

PER SERVING

Calories 159	Cholesterol 60 mg	DIETARY EXCHANGES:
Total Fat 4.0 g	Sodium 63 mg	½ other carbohydrate
Saturated Fat 1.0 g	Carbohydrates 6 g	3 lean meat
Trans Fat 0.0 g	Fiber 0 g	
Polyunsaturated Fat 0.5 g	Sugars 4 g	
Monounsaturated Fat 2.0 g	Protein 22 g	

Ham and Rice Croquettes

Serves 4

This comforting main dish is a great way to use up leftover rice. But if you don't have any, it's worth making a fresh batch. Add a southern accent with Sautéed Greens and Cabbage (page 261) or Oven-Fried Green Tomatoes with Poppy Seeds (page 269).

CROQUETTES

⅔ cup uncooked brown rice

1 small zucchini, shredded

½ cup diced red bell pepper

4 large egg whites

2 ounces lower-sodium, low-fat ham, all visible fat discarded, diced

¼ cup whole-wheat panko (Japanese-style bread crumbs)

2 medium green onions, thinly sliced

2 tablespoons shredded or grated Parmesan cheese

1 tablespoon Dijon mustard (lowest sodium available)

⅛ teaspoon salt

⅛ teaspoon pepper

. . . .

1 teaspoon canola or corn oil and 1 teaspoon canola or corn oil, divided use

Cooking spray

Prepare the rice using the package directions, omitting the salt and margarine.

In a medium bowl, using your hands or a spoon, combine the cooked rice and the remaining croquette ingredients.

In a large nonstick skillet, heat 1 teaspoon oil over medium heat, swirling to coat the bottom. Spoon eight ¼-cup mounds of the rice mixture (about half) into the skillet. Flatten slightly with a spatula. Lightly spray the top of the croquettes with cooking spray. Cook for 4 to 5 minutes on each side, or until browned. Transfer to a plate. Repeat with the remaining oil and croquette mixture, and more cooking spray.

COOK'S TIP: Use a mandoline to shred the zucchini for this recipe. The mandoline is a hand-operated kitchen device that makes short work of slicing, dicing, shredding, or grating firm vegetables and fruits. It has a sturdy rectangular frame and comes with a number of moveable blades that can be adjusted to cut in a variety of thicknesses. You can find mandolines in most housewares departments and kitchen specialty stores.

COOK'S TIP: These croquettes are easily reheated in a microwave. Put 4 croquettes on a microwaveable plate. Microwave on 100 percent power (high) for 1 to 2 minutes, or until heated through.

PER SERVING

Calories 207	Cholesterol 8 mg	DIETARY EXCHANGES:
Total Fat 4.0 g	Sodium 381 mg	2 starch
Saturated Fat 1.0 g	Carbohydrates 32 g	1 lean meat
Trans Fat 0.0 g	Fiber 4 g	
Polyunsaturated Fat 1.0 g	Sugars 3 g	
Monounsaturated Fat 1.5 g	Protein 11 g	

Pork with Corn-Cilantro Pesto

Serves 4 (plus about ½ cup pesto remaining)

The delicious pesto inside these pork pinwheels is a southwestern rendition of an Italian favorite. The recipe makes more pesto than you need for the pork, so try some of the extra with pasta or stir a dollop into soup, such as Rustic Tomato Soup (page 66) or Country-Style Vegetable Soup (page 55), for a fresh flavor boost.

Cooking spray

PESTO

- 1 **cup tightly packed fresh cilantro**
- ⅓ **cup no-salt-added whole-kernel corn, drained if canned or thawed if frozen**
- ¼ **cup tightly packed fresh parsley**
- ¼ **cup shredded or grated Parmesan or Romano cheese**
- 2 **tablespoons chopped pecans**
- 1 **tablespoon chopped shallot**
- 1 **tablespoon fresh lime juice (plus more if needed)**
- 2 **medium garlic cloves, quartered**
- ¼ **teaspoon salt**
- 1 **tablespoon plus 1 teaspoon olive oil**

. . . .

- 1 **1-pound pork tenderloin, all visible fat discarded**

SAUCE

- ½ **cup chopped onion**
- 1 **medium garlic clove, minced**
- 1 **8-ounce can no-salt-added tomato sauce**
- ¼ **teaspoon sugar**
- ¼ **teaspoon salt**
- ⅛ **teaspoon pepper**

Preheat the oven to 425°F. Lightly spray a shallow roasting pan and a wire rack or the broiler pan and rack with cooking spray.

In a food processor or blender, process the pesto ingredients except the oil until well combined, scraping the side as necessary. With the processor running, gradually pour in the oil. Process until well combined. If the pesto is thicker than you like, gradually add lime juice or water as needed.

Using a sharp knife, butterfly the pork. Starting at the top of the widest edge, cut the pork almost in half parallel to your work surface (through the middle of the meat), stopping about ½ inch from the opposite edge so the two halves are still joined. Open the split pork like a book. Using the smooth side of a meat mallet, lightly pound the pork to a thickness of ¼ inch, being careful not to tear it.

Spread ¼ cup pesto over the cut surface of the pork. (Cover and refrigerate the remaining pesto for another use.) Roll up the pork from a short end. Tie in several places with kitchen twine to keep the filling in place. Put the pork on the rack.

Roast for 20 minutes. Turn over the pork. Roast for 10 to 20 minutes, or until the pork registers 145°F on an instant-read thermometer. Transfer the pork to a cutting board. Let stand for 3 minutes. Discard the twine. Cut the pork crosswise into slices.

Meanwhile, lightly spray a medium saucepan with cooking spray. Cook the onion and minced garlic over medium heat for 3 to 4 minutes, or until the onion is soft, stirring occasionally.

Stir in the remaining sauce ingredients. Increase the heat to high and bring to a boil. Reduce the heat and simmer for 5 minutes, or until the desired consistency. Serve with the pork.

PER SERVING

Calories 179	Cholesterol 61 mg	DIETARY EXCHANGES:
Total Fat 6.0 g	Sodium 278 mg	2 vegetable
Saturated Fat 1.5 g	Carbohydrates 8 g	3 lean meat
Trans Fat 0.0 g	Fiber 2 g	
Polyunsaturated Fat 1.0 g	Sugars 4 g	
Monounsaturated Fat 3.0 g	Protein 23 g	

Spicy Baked Pork Chops

Serves 4

This crisp-coated pork dish cooks in less than half an hour, and the assembly-line preparation makes getting the chops ready a snap. For a quick side dish, try Sautéed Greens and Cabbage (page 261) or Apple-Lemon Carrots (page 255).

Cooking spray
¼ cup egg substitute
2 tablespoons fat-free milk
⅓ cup cornflake crumbs
2 tablespoons cornmeal
½ teaspoon dried marjoram, crumbled
⅛ teaspoon pepper
⅛ teaspoon dry mustard
⅛ teaspoon ground ginger
⅛ teaspoon cayenne
4 boneless pork loin chops (about 4 ounces each), all visible fat discarded

Preheat the oven to 375°F. Lightly spray a large shallow baking dish with cooking spray.

In a medium shallow bowl, whisk together the egg substitute and milk. In a shallow dish, such as a pie pan, stir together the crumbs, cornmeal, marjoram, pepper, mustard, ginger, and cayenne. Put the bowl, dish, and baking dish in a row, assembly-line fashion. Dip the pork in the egg substitute mixture, then in the crumb mixture, turning to coat at each step and gently shaking off any excess. Using your fingertips, gently press the coating so it adheres to the pork. Transfer the pork to the baking dish, arranging it in a single layer.

Bake for 15 minutes. Turn over the pork. Bake for 10 minutes, or until the pork registers 145°F on an instant-read thermometer. Remove from the oven. Let stand for 3 minutes.

PER SERVING

Calories 176	Cholesterol 58 mg	DIETARY EXCHANGES:
Total Fat 5.0 g	Sodium 126 mg	½ starch
Saturated Fat 1.5 g	Carbohydrates 11 g	3 lean meat
Trans Fat 0.0 g	Fiber 0 g	
Polyunsaturated Fat 0.5 g	Sugars 1 g	
Monounsaturated Fat 2.0 g	Protein 21 g	

Skillet Pork Chops with Cinnamon-Apple Salsa

Serves 4

This easy-to-prepare dish is a delicious twist on the classic combination of pork chops and applesauce. What a tasty way to incorporate more fruit into your diet! And don't forget your veggies, too. Try Wilted Spinach (page 268) or steamed green beans or broccoli.

½ teaspoon dried thyme, crumbled

¼ teaspoon garlic powder

4 pork loin chops with bone (about 5 ounces each), all visible fat discarded

SALSA

8 ounces Granny Smith apples, finely chopped

4 dried plums with orange essence, finely chopped

1 tablespoon firmly packed dark brown sugar

½ teaspoon grated orange zest

2 tablespoons fresh orange juice

¼ teaspoon ground cinnamon

Sprinkle the thyme and garlic powder over both sides of the pork.

In a large nonstick skillet, cook the pork over medium heat for 5 minutes on each side, or until it registers 145°F on an instant-read thermometer. Remove from the heat. Let stand for 3 minutes.

Meanwhile, in a medium serving bowl, gently stir together the salsa ingredients until well combined. Serve with the pork.

PER SERVING

Calories 206	Cholesterol 63 mg	DIETARY EXCHANGES:
Total Fat 5.5 g	Sodium 44 mg	1 fruit
Saturated Fat 1.5 g	Carbohydrates 19 g	3 lean meat
Trans Fat 0.0 g	Fiber 2 g	
Polyunsaturated Fat 0.5 g	Sugars 13 g	
Monounsaturated Fat 2.0 g	Protein 20 g	

Pork and Pepper Stew

Serves 4

This dish is traditionally served with baked or boiled potatoes, but you can also ladle it over fluffy brown rice or another whole grain, such as quinoa or farro.

Cooking spray
1 small red bell pepper, chopped
1 small yellow bell pepper, chopped
½ cup chopped onion
1 medium garlic clove, minced
1 pound pork tenderloin, all visible fat discarded, cut into ½-inch cubes
1 tablespoon all-purpose flour
2½ cups fat-free, low-sodium chicken broth
1 teaspoon grated orange zest
½ teaspoon ground coriander
¼ teaspoon salt
⅛ to ¼ teaspoon cayenne

Lightly spray a Dutch oven or large saucepan with cooking spray. Heat over medium heat. Cook the bell peppers, onion, and garlic for 10 minutes, or until the bell peppers are tender and the onion is very soft, stirring occasionally. Transfer to a bowl.

Increase the heat to medium high. Cook half the pork for about 5 minutes, or until browned on all sides, stirring frequently (the pork won't be done at this point). Transfer to a plate. Repeat with the remaining pork. Return all the pork to the Dutch oven.

Stir in the flour. Stir the vegetables and the remaining ingredients into the pork mixture. Increase the heat to high and bring to a boil. Reduce the heat and simmer, covered, for 20 minutes, or until the pork is tender, stirring occasionally.

PER SERVING

Calories 152	Cholesterol 60 mg	DIETARY EXCHANGES:
Total Fat 3.0 g	Sodium 210 mg	1 vegetable
Saturated Fat 1.0 g	Carbohydrates 6 g	3 lean meat
Trans Fat 0.0 g	Fiber 1 g	
Polyunsaturated Fat 0.5 g	Sugars 2 g	
Monounsaturated Fat 1.0 g	Protein 24 g	

Vegetarian Entrées

GRILLED PIZZA WITH GRILLED VEGETABLES 212

PASTA E FAGIOLI 214

PUMPKIN GNOCCHI 216

SOBA LO MEIN WITH EDAMAME AND VEGETABLES 218

PASTA WITH FRESH VEGETABLE SAUCE 220

GRILLED PORTOBELLO MUSHROOMS WITH COUSCOUS AND GREENS 222

POLENTA WITH SAUTÉED VEGETABLES 224

PAN-FRIED PASTA PANCAKE WITH VEGETABLES 226

SPAGHETTI WITH EGGPLANT SAUCE 227

BULGUR AND BUTTERNUT SQUASH 228

QUINOA IN VEGETABLE NESTS 229

GRILLED VEGETABLE QUESADILLAS 230

FIESTA BLACK BEAN NACHOS 232

SPINACH AND BLACK BEAN ENCHILADAS 233

EGGPLANT PARMIGIANA 234

SPICY LENTIL CURRY 236

THAI COCONUT CURRY WITH VEGETABLES 238

ROSEMARY-ARTICHOKE FRITTATA 240

WATERCRESS-CHEESE SOUFFLÉ 242

EDAMAME STIR-FRY 244

MEDITERRANEAN STRATA 245

Grilled Pizza with Grilled Vegetables

Serves 8

Making your own dough is worth the effort; prepare extra and freeze it for later use (see the Cook's Tip on page 213). You can also customize your pizzas by using whatever vegetables are in season.

DOUGH

- 1 cup lukewarm water (105°F to 115°F)
- 1 ¼-ounce package active dry yeast
- 1 teaspoon sugar
- 3 cups white whole-wheat flour, 3 to 4 tablespoons white whole-wheat flour, and ¼ cup white whole-wheat flour (if needed), divided use
- 2 tablespoons olive oil
- ⅛ teaspoon salt

. . . .

- Cooking spray
- 2 medium thin zucchini, sliced (about 2 cups)
- 2 medium red bell peppers
- 1 bunch of medium asparagus, trimmed (about 16 medium stalks)
- 1 large portobello mushroom
- Cornmeal for rolling out the dough
- 2 to 3 tablespoons no-salt-added tomato paste
- 8 large fresh basil leaves, coarsely chopped
- 1¼ cups shredded low-fat mozzarella cheese

In a small bowl, combine the water, yeast, and sugar, stirring to dissolve. Let stand for 5 minutes.

Meanwhile, in a large bowl, stir together 3 cups flour, the oil, and salt.

When the yeast is ready, add it to the flour mixture, stirring until the dough starts to pull away from the side of the bowl.

Using 3 to 4 tablespoons flour, lightly flour a flat surface. Turn out the dough. Knead for 5 minutes, gradually adding, if needed, enough of the remaining ¼ cup flour to make the dough smooth and elastic. (It shouldn't be dry or stick to the surface. You may not need any of the additional ¼ cup flour, or you may need the entire amount if the dough is too sticky.)

Lightly spray a separate large bowl and a piece of plastic wrap large enough to cover the top of the bowl with cooking spray.

Transfer the dough to the bowl, turning to coat with the cooking spray. Cover the bowl with the plastic wrap with the sprayed side down. Let the dough rise in a warm, draft-free place (about 85°F) for about 1 hour, or until doubled in bulk.

Meanwhile, lightly spray the grill rack with cooking spray. Preheat the grill on medium high.

Grill the zucchini, bell peppers, asparagus, and mushroom for 15 to 20 minutes, or until the peppers are blackened and the other vegetables are tender and well marked, turning the peppers to char evenly and turning the other vegetables after 10 minutes.

Transfer the peppers to a large bowl. Cover with plastic wrap. Let stand for 20 to 30 minutes, or until cool enough to handle. Cut off the asparagus tips, reserving the stalks for another use. Slice the mushroom. Transfer the zucchini, asparagus tips, and mushroom to a medium plate.

When the peppers have cooled, cut them in half. Discard the stems, ribs, and seeds. Using your fingers, paper towels, or a knife, gently peel them, discarding the skin. Slice the peppers. Transfer to the plate with the vegetables.

Sprinkle the cornmeal on a flat surface. Transfer the dough to the surface and punch it down. Divide into four equal pieces. Roll each piece of dough into an 8-inch circle, keeping them about ¼ inch thick.

Grill the dough, covered, with the cornmeal sides up for 4 minutes, or until the other sides are lightly browned. Remove from the grill. Using a pastry brush, coat the grilled sides with the tomato paste, rubbing it into the surface. Top with the vegetables. Sprinkle the basil and mozzarella over the vegetables.

Grill for 5 to 6 minutes, or until the mozzarella is melted. Remove from the grill. Let stand for about 2 minutes before serving.

....

COOK'S TIP: If you decide to make extra pizza dough to freeze, roll it into a mound and flatten it slightly. Lightly spray an airtight freezer bag with cooking spray. Transfer the dough to the bag and seal tightly. Freeze the dough for up to three months. When you need it, thaw it in the refrigerator for at least 8 hours. Then let it come to room temperature, 1 to 2 hours, before rolling it out and making the pizza as directed.

....

PER SERVING

Calories 262	Cholesterol 6 mg	DIETARY EXCHANGES:
Total Fat 6.0 g	Sodium 171 mg	2 starch
Saturated Fat 1.0 g	Carbohydrates 37 g	1 vegetable
Trans Fat 0.0 g	Fiber 8 g	½ lean meat
Polyunsaturated Fat 1.0 g	Sugars 6 g	½ fat
Monounsaturated Fat 3.5 g	Protein 14 g	

Pasta e Fagioli

Serves 8

The traditional Italian soup of pasta and beans is lightened up in this recipe. Serve it warm in the winter and cold in the summer. For unlimited possibilities, experiment with different beans, pasta, and herbs every time you make this dish.

- 2 teaspoons olive oil
- 1 large sweet onion, such as Vidalia, Maui, or Oso Sweet, chopped
- 1 cup finely chopped celery
- 3 medium garlic cloves, minced, or 1½ teaspoons bottled minced garlic
- 1 cup diced mushrooms
- ¾ cup no-salt-added canned navy beans, rinsed and drained
- ¾ cup no-salt-added canned fava beans, rinsed and drained
- ¾ cup no-salt-added canned chickpeas, rinsed and drained
- ½ cup medium-dry white wine (regular or nonalcoholic) or fat-free, low-sodium vegetable broth
- 5 oil-packed sun-dried tomatoes, drained well and finely chopped
- ¼ cup balsamic vinegar
- 3 medium dried bay leaves
- 1 tablespoon dried oregano, crumbled
- 1 teaspoon dried basil, crumbled
- ¼ to ½ teaspoon crushed red pepper flakes, or to taste
- 1 pound dried whole-grain pasta (ziti preferred)
- ½ cup chopped fresh parsley
- ¼ cup shredded or grated Parmesan cheese and ½ cup shredded or grated Parmesan cheese (Parmigiano-Reggiano preferred), divided use

In a stockpot, heat the oil over medium-high heat, swirling to coat the bottom. Cook the onion, celery, and garlic for 3 minutes, or until the onion is soft, stirring frequently.

Stir in the mushrooms, navy and fava beans, chickpeas, wine, tomatoes, vinegar, bay leaves, oregano, and basil. Increase the heat to high and bring to a boil.

Stir in the red pepper flakes. Reduce the heat and simmer, covered, for 10 minutes, stirring occasionally. Discard the bay leaves.

Meanwhile, prepare the pasta using the package directions, omitting the salt. Drain well in a colander.

Transfer the pasta to a large bowl. Add the onion mixture, parsley, and ¼ cup Parmesan, stirring to combine. Just before serving, sprinkle with the remaining ½ cup Parmesan.

PER SERVING

Calories 340	Cholesterol 5 mg	DIETARY EXCHANGES:
Total Fat 5.5 g	Sodium 162 mg	4 starch
Saturated Fat 1.5 g	Carbohydrates 59 g	½ lean meat
Trans Fat 0.0 g	Fiber 10 g	
Polyunsaturated Fat 1.0 g	Sugars 6 g	
Monounsaturated Fat 2.0 g	Protein 15 g	

Pumpkin Gnocchi

Serves 4

Most gnocchi available in the United States are made with potato, but creamy, slightly sweet pumpkin adds a delicious twist to the pillowy morsels, which are complemented by savory green beans and a silky sauce.

8 ounces frozen Italian-cut green beans
1 cup canned solid-pack pumpkin (not pie filling)
½ cup egg substitute
¼ teaspoon pepper
2 cups white whole-wheat flour and 2 to 3 tablespoons white whole-wheat flour, divided use

SAUCE

1 cup fat-free half-and-half
1½ tablespoons all-purpose flour
¼ cup shredded or grated Parmesan cheese
1 teaspoon grated lemon zest
¼ teaspoon pepper
⅛ teaspoon salt

Prepare the green beans using the package directions, omitting the salt and margarine.

Drain well in a colander. Cover to keep warm. Set aside.

Meanwhile, in a medium bowl, whisk together the pumpkin, egg substitute, and ¼ teaspoon pepper.

Add 2 cups flour to the pumpkin mixture, stirring just until the flour is combined but no flour is visible and the dough forms a ball. Don't overmix or the dough may become gummy.

Fill a stockpot with water. Bring to a simmer over high heat.

Divide the dough into 4 equal pieces. Lightly flour a flat surface with 2 to 3 tablespoons flour. Using your hands, lightly roll each piece of the dough into a 12-inch-long cylinder. Cut each cylinder crosswise into 24 pieces. If desired, use a fork to slightly flatten each piece and create grooves, which help hold the sauce.

Put half the gnocchi in the simmering water. After the pieces float to the surface (about 1 minute), cook for 3 to 4 minutes, or until tender and cooked through (when cut in half, they shouldn't look chalky, which indicates uncooked flour), stirring occasionally. Using a slotted spoon, transfer the gnocchi to a medium bowl. Cover to keep warm. Repeat with the remaining gnocchi.

Meanwhile, in a small saucepan, whisk together the half-and-half and the remaining 1½ tablespoons flour. The mixture will be slightly lumpy. Bring to a simmer over medium-high heat, whisking occasionally. Simmer for 1 to 2 minutes, or until thickened, whisking occasionally. Remove from the heat.

Stir in the remaining sauce ingredients.

Spoon the gnocchi into serving bowls. Spoon the green beans over the gnocchi. Ladle the sauce over all.

PER SERVING

Calories 370	Cholesterol 4 mg	DIETARY EXCHANGES:
Total Fat 2.5 g	Sodium 422 mg	4 starch
Saturated Fat 1.0 g	Carbohydrates 71 g	2 vegetable
Trans Fat 0.0 g	Fiber 6 g	1 lean meat
Polyunsaturated Fat 0.5 g	Sugars 8 g	
Monounsaturated Fat 0.5 g	Protein 18 g	

Soba Lo Mein with Edamame and Vegetables

Serves 4

The secret to success for this dish is not to overcook the soba, thin Japanese noodles made from buckwheat flour. The noodles have a strong nutty flavor that's a perfect foil for the Asian-inspired sauce. Edamame adds protein, while lightly cooked vegetables add crunch and color.

- 1½ cups frozen shelled edamame
- 4 ounces dried soba noodles

SAUCE
- ¼ cup fat-free, low-sodium vegetable broth
- 2 tablespoons hoisin sauce (lowest sodium available)
- 1 tablespoon soy sauce (lowest sodium available)
- 1 teaspoon sugar (optional)

....

- 1 teaspoon canola or corn oil
- 2 medium garlic cloves, minced
- 2 medium carrots, thinly sliced
- 4 ounces sugar snap peas, trimmed
- 2 medium stalks bok choy, stems and leaves thinly sliced
- ½ medium onion, thinly sliced

Prepare the edamame using the package directions, omitting the salt. Drain well in a colander. Set aside.

Prepare the noodles using the package directions, omitting the salt. Drain well in a colander. Set aside.

In a small bowl, whisk together the sauce ingredients. Set aside.

In a large nonstick skillet, heat the oil over medium-high heat, swirling to coat the bottom. Cook the garlic for 15 seconds, stirring constantly. Watch carefully so it doesn't burn. Stir in the carrots and peas. Cook for 1 minute, stirring constantly. Stir in the bok choy and onion. Cook for 1 to 2 minutes, or until the vegetables are tender-crisp, stirring constantly.

Stir in the edamame, noodles, and sauce. Cook for 1 minute, or until the mixture is heated through, stirring constantly.

COOK'S TIP ON BOK CHOY: Both the crunchy white stems and the delicate leafy green part of bok choy are edible. Cook the stems or eat them raw like celery. Cook the green parts as you would spinach. Both stems and greens are good stir-fried or added to soups (the greens cook quickly, so add them near the end of the cooking time).

PER SERVING

Calories 230	Cholesterol 0 mg	DIETARY EXCHANGES:
Total Fat 4.0 g	Sodium 209 mg	2 starch
Saturated Fat 0.0 g	Carbohydrates 38 g	2 vegetable
Trans Fat 0.0 g	Fiber 7 g	1 lean meat
Polyunsaturated Fat 1.5 g	Sugars 11 g	
Monounsaturated Fat 2.0 g	Protein 13 g	

Pasta with Fresh Vegetable Sauce

Serves 6

Long, slow simmering yields a rich, deeply flavored sauce that is sopped up beautifully by whole-grain pasta. The sauce tastes even better the next day, so if you have the time, prepare it ahead.

Cooking spray

SAUCE

1 teaspoon olive oil

1 large red or white onion, chopped

6 medium green onions, chopped

4 medium garlic cloves, minced

1 15.5-ounce can no-salt-added kidney beans, rinsed and drained

1 14.5-ounce can no-salt-added tomatoes, undrained

8 ounces button mushrooms, sliced

2 medium red, green, or yellow bell peppers, or any combination, chopped

2 medium ribs of celery with leaves, chopped

1 cup water

½ cup dry red wine (regular or nonalcoholic) (optional)

¼ cup finely chopped fresh parsley

1 tablespoon chopped fresh oregano or 1 teaspoon dried oregano, crumbled

1 tablespoon chopped fresh basil or ½ teaspoon dried basil, crumbled

1 medium dried bay leaf

Pepper to taste

. . . .

12 ounces dried whole-grain pasta, such as spaghetti

1 cup shredded low-fat mozzarella cheese

Lightly spray a large saucepan or Dutch oven with cooking spray. Heat the oil over medium-high heat, swirling to coat the bottom. Cook the red onion, green onions, and garlic for about 3 minutes, or until soft, stirring frequently.

Stir in the remaining sauce ingredients, including the tomatoes with liquid. Increase the heat to high and bring to a boil. Reduce the heat and simmer, covered, for 1 hour, stirring frequently. Discard the bay leaf.

Meanwhile, prepare the pasta using the package directions, omitting the salt. Drain well in a colander. Transfer to plates.

Just before serving, sprinkle the pasta with the mozzarella. Ladle the sauce over all.

PER SERVING

Calories 372	Cholesterol 7 mg	DIETARY EXCHANGES:
Total Fat 3.5 g	Sodium 192 mg	4 starch
Saturated Fat 1.0 g	Carbohydrates 68 g	2 vegetable
Trans Fat 0.0 g	Fiber 14 g	1 lean meat
Polyunsaturated Fat 0.5 g	Sugars 10 g	
Monounsaturated Fat 1.5 g	Protein 20 g	

Grilled Portobello Mushrooms with Couscous and Greens

Serves 4

The grand size and meaty texture of the portobello mushroom make it a perfect base for fluffy couscous and vibrant greens. Crumbled feta cheese adds protein and a burst of tangy flavor.

    4 medium portobello mushrooms, stems discarded
    ¼ cup balsamic vinegar
       Cooking spray
    ½ cup fat-free, low-sodium vegetable broth
    ½ cup water and 2 tablespoons water, divided use
    ¼ teaspoon ground turmeric
    ⅔ cup uncooked whole-wheat couscous
    ¼ cup sweetened dried cranberries
    ½ teaspoon grated lemon zest
    ⅛ teaspoon salt
    1 teaspoon olive oil
    2 medium garlic cloves, minced
    6 ounces collard greens or kale or 8 ounces spinach, chopped
    1 tablespoon light tub margarine
    ½ medium red bell pepper, finely chopped
    2 ounces fat-free feta cheese, crumbled

On the smooth side of each mushroom, cut four slits, each 2 to 3 inches long and about ½ inch deep. In a 13 x 9 x 2-inch glass baking dish, arrange the mushrooms in a single layer with the smooth side up.

Sprinkle half the vinegar over the mushrooms. Lightly spray with cooking spray. Turn over the mushrooms. Sprinkle the remaining vinegar over the mushrooms. Lightly spray with cooking spray. Cover and refrigerate until needed (up to 1 hour).

In a medium saucepan, bring the broth, ½ cup water, and the turmeric to a boil over high heat.

Stir in the couscous, cranberries, lemon zest, and salt. Remove from the heat. Let stand, covered, for at least 5 minutes. Fluff with a fork.

Meanwhile, lightly spray a grill rack with cooking spray. Preheat the grill on medium high.

In a medium saucepan, heat the oil over medium heat, swirling to coat the bottom. Cook the garlic for 1 minute, stirring occasionally.

Stir in the greens and the remaining 2 tablespoons water. Cook, covered, for 2 to 3 minutes, or until the greens are tender.

Add the margarine. Stir for 30 seconds, or until melted. Remove from the heat. Cover to keep warm.

Grill the mushrooms for 2 to 3 minutes on each side, or until tender.

Transfer the mushrooms to plates with the stem side up. Spoon the couscous over each mushroom. Spoon the greens over the couscous. Sprinkle with the bell pepper and feta.

COOK'S TIP: The couscous mixture and cooked greens can be covered and refrigerated separately for up to five days. To reheat each part, microwave them in a microwaveable container on 100 percent power (high) for 1 to 2 minutes.

PER SERVING

Calories 217	Cholesterol 0 mg	DIETARY EXCHANGES:
Total Fat 3.0 g	Sodium 371 mg	1½ starch
Saturated Fat 0.0 g	Carbohydrates 39 g	2 vegetable
Trans Fat 0.0 g	Fiber 5 g	½ other carbohydrate
Polyunsaturated Fat 0.5 g	Sugars 11 g	½ lean meat
Monounsaturated Fat 1.5 g	Protein 9 g	

Polenta with Sautéed Vegetables

Serves 4

Creamy, homemade polenta forms a perfect bed for summertime vegetables that have been simmered in a well-spiced tomato sauce. A sprinkle of Parmesan provides the final flourish.

1 tablespoon olive oil

2 medium garlic cloves, minced

1 medium eggplant (about 1 pound), diced

1 small yellow summer squash (about 4 ounces), thinly sliced

1 small zucchini (about 4 ounces), thinly sliced

1 medium red bell pepper, cut into ½-inch strips

1 8-ounce can no-salt-added tomato sauce

½ cup fat-free, low-sodium vegetable broth

1 teaspoon dried oregano, crumbled

¼ teaspoon salt

¼ teaspoon pepper

POLENTA

1 cup fat-free, low-sodium vegetable broth

1 cup fat-free milk

½ cup yellow cornmeal (coarse-grained for more robust texture, fine-grained for creamier texture)

. . . .

¼ cup shredded or grated Parmesan cheese

In a large nonstick skillet, heat the oil over medium-high heat, swirling to coat the bottom. Cook the garlic for 10 seconds, stirring constantly. Watch carefully so it doesn't burn.

Stir in the eggplant, summer squash, zucchini, and bell pepper. Cook for 5 to 6 minutes, or until tender, stirring occasionally. Add water, 1 tablespoon at a time, if the mixture begins to stick to the skillet.

Stir in the tomato sauce, ½ cup broth, the oregano, salt, and pepper. Bring to a simmer. Reduce the heat and simmer, partially covered, for 15 minutes.

Meanwhile, in a medium saucepan, bring the remaining 1 cup broth and the milk to a simmer over medium-high heat. Reduce the heat to medium. Using a long-handled whisk, carefully whisk the mixture to create a swirl. Slowly pour the cornmeal in a steady stream into the swirl, whisking constantly. After all the cornmeal is added, hold the pan steady and continue whisking for 1 to 2 minutes, or until the polenta is the desired consistency.

Spoon the polenta into bowls. Spoon the vegetables on top. Sprinkle with the Parmesan.

....

COOK'S TIP ON PARMESAN CHEESE: For this and other recipes calling for Parmesan cheese, you may want to buy a wedge of the cheese and shave the specified amount as you need it. A potato peeler or box grater works well for this. For a real taste treat, try Parmigiano-Reggiano, a pricey Italian import that practically melts in your mouth.

....

PER SERVING

		DIETARY EXCHANGES:
Calories 203	Cholesterol 5 mg	
Total Fat 5.5 g	Sodium 278 mg	1 starch
Saturated Fat 1.5 g	Carbohydrates 33 g	3 vegetable
Trans Fat 0.0 g	Fiber 6 g	½ lean meat
Polyunsaturated Fat 0.5 g	Sugars 12 g	1 fat
Monounsaturated Fat 3.0 g	Protein 9 g	

Pan-Fried Pasta Pancake with Vegetables

Serves 4

This dish is a great way to use up leftover cooked pasta, which gets brown and crisp as it cooks. Serve it in wedges, with a leafy green salad on the side.

8 ounces dried whole-grain pasta, such as linguine, vermicelli, or spaghetti (or 4 cups cooked pasta)

1 medium carrot, shredded

2 medium green onions, thinly sliced

½ cup snow peas, trimmed and cut into ½-inch pieces

1 teaspoon toasted sesame oil

1 teaspoon canola or corn oil

1 cup egg substitute

¼ teaspoon salt

⅛ teaspoon pepper

Prepare the pasta using the package directions, omitting the salt. Drain well in a colander. Transfer to a large bowl. Refrigerate for at least 10 minutes.

Stir the carrot, green onions, peas, and sesame oil into the cooled pasta.

In a medium nonstick skillet, heat the canola oil over medium heat, swirling to coat the bottom. Spread the pasta mixture in the bottom of the pan. Cook for 1 minute without stirring. Reduce the heat to low.

In a small bowl, whisk together the egg substitute, salt, and pepper. Pour over the pasta, tilting the pan to distribute the egg mixture. Don't stir.

Cook, covered, for 10 to 12 minutes, or until cooked through. To brown the other side, invert the pancake onto a plate and slide it back into the pan. Cook for 1 to 2 minutes.

COOK'S TIP: A pizza cutter works well for slicing this pancake into wedges.

PER SERVING

Calories 265	Cholesterol 0 mg	DIETARY EXCHANGES:
Total Fat 3.0 g	Sodium 290 mg	3 starch
Saturated Fat 0.5 g	Carbohydrates 47 g	1 vegetable
Trans Fat 0.0 g	Fiber 8 g	1 lean meat
Polyunsaturated Fat 1.0 g	Sugars 5 g	
Monounsaturated Fat 1.5 g	Protein 15 g	

Spaghetti with Eggplant Sauce

Serves 6

The Italian name for this dish is *melanzana affogate,* or "suffocated eggplant," because the eggplant becomes so soft that it "melts" into the tomato sauce. Serve with a spinach salad with Parmesan-Peppercorn Ranch Dressing (page 100).

SAUCE

- 3 tablespoons olive oil
- 1 medium eggplant, peeled and cubed
- 1 medium onion, sliced
- 1 medium green bell pepper, sliced
- 1 medium garlic clove, minced
- 1 cup chopped Italian plum (Roma) tomatoes
- 1 cup no-salt-added tomato juice
- 2 teaspoons dried basil, crumbled
- 1 teaspoon dried oregano, crumbled

. . . .

- 12 ounces dried whole-grain spaghetti
- ¼ cup plus 2 tablespoons shredded or grated Parmesan cheese

In a large skillet or stockpot, heat the oil over medium-high heat, swirling to coat the bottom. Cook the eggplant for 10 minutes, stirring frequently. Stir in the onion, bell pepper, and garlic. Cook for 3 to 5 minutes, or until the eggplant is very soft (almost mushy), stirring occasionally.

Stir in the remaining sauce ingredients. Reduce the heat and simmer, covered, for 30 to 40 minutes, or until the eggplant is broken down, stirring occasionally.

Meanwhile, prepare the pasta using the package directions, omitting the salt. Drain well in a colander. Add the pasta to the sauce, stirring to coat. Just before serving, sprinkle with the Parmesan.

PER SERVING		
Calories 331	Cholesterol 4 mg	DIETARY EXCHANGES:
Total Fat 10.0 g	Sodium 118 mg	3 starch
Saturated Fat 2.0 g	Carbohydrates 53 g	2 vegetable
Trans Fat 0.0 g	Fiber 10 g	1½ fat
Polyunsaturated Fat 1.0 g	Sugars 9 g	
Monounsaturated Fat 6.0 g	Protein 11 g	

Bulgur and Butternut Squash

Serves 4

Nutty bulgur is an ideal complement to tender butternut squash. Using frozen squash means you can enjoy this dish any time of year.

- 1 cup fat-free, low-sodium vegetable broth
- ½ cup uncooked instant, or fine-grain, bulgur
- 2 teaspoons olive oil
- 1 medium red bell pepper, chopped
- 1 medium onion, chopped
- 20 ounces frozen diced butternut squash, thawed
- ¼ teaspoon salt
- ¼ teaspoon pepper
- 2 tablespoons balsamic vinegar
- 1 tablespoon light brown sugar
- 1 tablespoon Dijon mustard (lowest sodium available)
- ¼ cup chopped pecans, dry-roasted

In a medium saucepan, bring the broth to a simmer over medium-high heat. Stir in the bulgur. Reduce the heat and simmer, covered, for 15 minutes, or until the broth is absorbed. Remove from the heat. Let stand for 5 minutes. Fluff with a fork.

Meanwhile, in a large nonstick skillet, heat the oil over medium-high heat, swirling to coat the bottom. Cook the bell pepper and onion for 3 to 4 minutes, or until the bell pepper is tender and the onion is soft, stirring frequently. Stir in the squash, salt, and pepper. Cook for 4 to 5 minutes, or until heated through, stirring gently if you want the squash to stay chunky (no need to be careful if you want the squash more mashed).

In a small microwaveable bowl, whisk together the vinegar, brown sugar, and mustard. Microwave on 100 percent power (high) for 15 to 20 seconds, or until heated through. Transfer to a small serving bowl.

Spoon the bulgur into serving bowls. Spoon the squash mixture over the bulgur. Sprinkle with the pecans. Serve the sauce on the side.

PER SERVING

Calories 303	Cholesterol 0 mg	DIETARY EXCHANGES:
Total Fat 13 g	Sodium 239 mg	2½ starch
Saturated Fat 1 g	Carbohydrates 46 g	1 vegetable
Trans Fat 0 g	Fiber 8 g	2 fat
Polyunsaturated Fat 3 g	Sugars 13 g	
Monounsaturated Fat 7 g	Protein 7 g	

Quinoa in Vegetable Nests

Serves 4

Crunchy, thinly sliced vegetables make colorful nests for delicate quinoa studded with pecans and flavored with Asian flair.

    1   cup uncooked quinoa, rinsed and drained
    1½ cups shredded napa cabbage
    1   cup thinly sliced red cabbage
    2   medium carrots, cut into very thin strips
    ½   medium yellow bell pepper, cut into very thin strips
    ¼   cup chopped pecans, dry-roasted
    2   teaspoons fresh lime juice
    2   teaspoons plain rice vinegar
    2   teaspoons soy sauce (lowest sodium available)
    1   medium garlic clove, minced
    ⅛   teaspoon pepper
    2   medium green onions, halved crosswise and cut into
        very thin strips

Prepare the quinoa using the package directions, omitting the salt. Transfer to a medium bowl. Fluff with a fork. Cover and refrigerate for at least 30 minutes.

Meanwhile, in a medium bowl, stir together the napa cabbage, red cabbage, carrots, and bell pepper.

Stir the remaining ingredients except the green onions into the cooled quinoa.

Spoon the cabbage mixture into shallow bowls. Make a "nest" in the center of the vegetables. Spoon the quinoa mixture into the nests. Sprinkle with the green onions.

....

COOK'S TIP ON QUINOA: Often called a supergrain because of the amount of protein and other nutrients it contains, quinoa is actually the fruit of a plant related to spinach, Swiss chard, and beets.

....

PER SERVING

Calories 242	Cholesterol 0 mg	DIETARY EXCHANGES:
Total Fat 7.5 g	Sodium 103 mg	2 starch
Saturated Fat 0.5 g	Carbohydrates 37 g	1 vegetable
Trans Fat 0.0 g	Fiber 6 g	1 fat
Polyunsaturated Fat 3.0 g	Sugars 6 g	
Monounsaturated Fat 3.5 g	Protein 8 g	

Grilled Vegetable Quesadillas

Serves 4

This summertime version includes grilled vegetables, which can come right from your backyard garden or local farmers' market. Enjoy these quesadillas with a salad of dark, leafy greens tossed with Gazpacho Dressing (page 99).

Cooking spray
1 medium ear of corn, husks and silk discarded
1 medium red bell pepper, halved lengthwise, seeds and ribs discarded
1 medium yellow summer squash, ends trimmed, halved lengthwise
½ small onion
¾ cup shredded low-fat 4-cheese Mexican blend
1 medium plum (Roma) tomato, diced
2 teaspoons fresh lime juice
¼ teaspoon chili powder
⅛ teaspoon pepper
4 6-inch corn tortillas
½ cup salsa (lowest sodium available)
½ cup fat-free sour cream

Lightly spray the grill rack with cooking spray. Preheat the grill on medium high.

Lightly spray the corn, bell pepper, squash, and onion with cooking spray.

Grill the corn for 2 minutes on each side. Grill the bell pepper, squash, and onion for 1 to 2 minutes on each side. Transfer to a cutting board. Let cool for 10 minutes. Dice the bell pepper, squash, and onion. Transfer to a medium bowl. Using a sharp knife, cut the corn kernels off the cob. Add to the bell pepper mixture.

Stir in the Mexican blend cheese, tomato, lime juice, chili powder, and pepper.

Heat a nonstick griddle or large cast-iron skillet over medium heat. Lightly spray one side of a tortilla with cooking spray. Put the tortilla on the griddle with the sprayed side down. Spread a heaping ⅓ cup vegetable mixture on half the tortilla. Fold the other half over the filling. Cook for 1 to 2 minutes on each side, or until the tortilla is golden brown and the cheese has melted. Transfer to a cutting board and cover to keep warm. Repeat with the remaining tortillas and filling.

Just before serving, cut each quesadilla in half. Top each piece with the salsa and sour cream.

....

COOK'S TIP ON CORN: To easily remove corn kernels from the cob, place one end of the corn cob in the hole in the center of a tube pan or Bundt pan. As you carefully cut downward along the cob, the corn kernels will fall into the pan.

....

PER SERVING

Calories 157	Cholesterol 10 mg	DIETARY EXCHANGES:
Total Fat 2.5 g	Sodium 303 mg	1½ starch
Saturated Fat 1.0 g	Carbohydrates 24 g	1 vegetable
Trans Fat 0.0 g	Fiber 3 g	1 lean meat
Polyunsaturated Fat 0.5 g	Sugars 8 g	
Monounsaturated Fat 0.5 g	Protein 10 g	

Fiesta Black Bean Nachos

Serves 4

This meatless entrée is quick to prepare and sure to become a family favorite. If you like spicier foods, sprinkle some fresh chopped jalapeños on top.

Cooking spray
4 **ounces no-salt-added baked tortilla chips (about 4 cups)**
1 **15.5-ounce can no-salt-added black beans, rinsed and drained**
½ **small red onion, diced**
½ **medium yellow bell pepper, diced**
16 **cherry tomatoes, halved**
1 **cup shredded low-fat Cheddar cheese**
¼ **cup fat-free sour cream**

Preheat the oven to 350°F. Lightly spray a large baking sheet with cooking spray.

Arrange the chips in a single layer on the baking sheet. Sprinkle with the beans, onion, bell pepper, tomatoes, and Cheddar.

Bake for 10 to 12 minutes, or until the nachos are heated through and the Cheddar is melted. Dollop each serving with the sour cream.

....

cook's tip: If you prefer, you can buy corn or whole-wheat tortillas and bake your own chips. Cut the tortillas into wedges. Arrange the wedges in a single layer on a large baking sheet. Bake at 350°F for 10 minutes, or until lightly golden.

....

PER SERVING

Calories 286	Cholesterol 8 mg	DIETARY EXCHANGES:
Total Fat 3.0 g	Sodium 191 mg	3 starch
Saturated Fat 1.5 g	Carbohydrates 48 g	2 lean meat
Trans Fat 0.0 g	Fiber 7 g	
Polyunsaturated Fat 0.5 g	Sugars 7 g	
Monounsaturated Fat 1.0 g	Protein 18 g	

Spinach and Black Bean Enchiladas

Earthy spinach and hearty black beans marry beautifully in these Mexican-inspired tortilla roll-ups. Sour cream spiked with lime juice makes a velvety topping, and the enchiladas are kissed with melted cheese.

- 1 **pound baby spinach or 10 ounces frozen leaf spinach**
  Cooking spray
- 1 **15.5-ounce can no-salt-added black beans, rinsed and drained**
- ½ **cup salsa (lowest sodium available)**
- ¼ **teaspoon ground cumin**
- ¼ **teaspoon chili powder**
- 6 **6-inch corn tortillas**
- ½ **cup fat-free sour cream**
- 1½ **to 2 teaspoons fresh lime juice**
- 1 **cup shredded low-fat Monterey Jack cheese**
- 2 **medium Italian plum (Roma) tomatoes, diced**
- 2 **medium green onions, thinly sliced**

In a soup pot or Dutch oven, bring several quarts of water to a boil over high heat. Cook the fresh spinach for 1 minute. Or prepare the frozen spinach using the package directions, omitting the salt and margarine. Drain well in a colander. Using the back of a spoon, press out the liquid.

Preheat the oven to 350°F. Lightly spray a medium shallow baking dish with cooking spray.

In a medium bowl, stir together the spinach, black beans, salsa, cumin, and chili powder. Place the tortillas on a work surface. Spoon the mixture down the center of each tortilla. Roll up jelly-roll style and place with the seam side down in the baking dish. Bake for 15 minutes.

Meanwhile, stir together the sour cream and lime juice.

Remove the cooked enchiladas from the oven. Spread the sour cream mixture over the top. Sprinkle with the Monterey Jack, tomatoes, and green onions. Bake for 5 minutes, or until the Monterey Jack is melted.

PER SERVING

Calories 199	Cholesterol 14 mg	DIETARY EXCHANGES:
Total Fat 4.0 g	Sodium 298 mg	1½ starch
Saturated Fat 2.0 g	Carbohydrates 27 g	1 vegetable
Trans Fat 0.0 g	Fiber 6 g	1 lean meat
Polyunsaturated Fat 0.5 g	Sugars 6 g	
Monounsaturated Fat 1.0 g	Protein 14 g	

Eggplant Parmigiana

Serves 6

Broiling the eggplant instead of frying it is the key to reducing the fat in this recipe, while tofu increases the protein. To complete the meal, add a garden salad with Creamy Herb Dressing (page 98) or Citrus-Tarragon Vinaigrette (page 102) and a crusty whole-grain roll.

SAUCE

- 2 8-ounce cans no-salt-added tomato sauce
- 9 ounces frozen artichoke hearts, thawed and drained
- 1 6-ounce can no-salt-added tomato paste
- 1 tablespoon dried Italian seasoning, crumbled
- 2 medium garlic cloves, minced
- 1 teaspoon olive oil
- ¼ teaspoon fennel seeds, crushed (optional)
- ⅛ teaspoon pepper

  Dash of red hot-pepper sauce
  ....

  Olive oil cooking spray
- 1 medium eggplant (about 1 pound), cut into ⅜-inch rounds
- 10 ounces light firm tofu, drained and patted dry
- 1 large egg white
- 1 cup shredded low-fat mozzarella cheese
- 1 tablespoon all-purpose flour
- ⅓ cup shredded or grated Parmesan cheese
- ⅓ cup plain dry bread crumbs (lowest sodium available)

In a food processor or blender, process the sauce ingredients for 30 seconds, or until no lumps remain. Pour into a medium bowl. Set aside.

Preheat the broiler.

Lightly spray a large baking sheet with cooking spray. Arrange the eggplant slices in a single layer on the baking sheet.

Broil about 4 inches from the heat for 3 to 4 minutes on each side. Watch carefully so it doesn't burn. Set the eggplant aside to let cool.

Preheat the oven to 350°F.

In a food processor or blender, process the tofu and egg white until smooth.

In a small bowl, toss the mozzarella with the flour to keep the mozzarella from clumping.

In an 11 x 7 x 2-inch glass baking dish, layer the ingredients as follows: one-third of the sauce, half the eggplant, one-third of the sauce, all the mozzarella mixture, all the tofu mixture, the remaining eggplant, the remaining sauce, the Parmesan, and the bread crumbs.

Bake for 35 minutes. Let stand for 5 minutes before serving.

PER SERVING

Calories 198	Cholesterol 11 mg	DIETARY EXCHANGES:
Total Fat 5.0 g	Sodium 345 mg	½ starch
Saturated Fat 2.0 g	Carbohydrates 26 g	4 vegetable
Trans Fat 0.0 g	Fiber 8 g	1½ lean meat
Polyunsaturated Fat 0.5 g	Sugars 10 g	
Monounsaturated Fat 2.0 g	Protein 15 g	

Spicy Lentil Curry

Serves 6

Serve this curry by itself or try it over brown rice with a dollop of fat-free plain yogurt topping each serving. For leftovers, spoon the curry into whole-grain pita pockets.

 6 cups water
 1½ cups dried lentils, sorted for stones and shriveled lentils, rinsed, and drained
 1 teaspoon cumin seeds or ground cumin
 1 large onion, chopped
 1 teaspoon canola or corn oil
 1 medium tomato, chopped
 1 medium red chile (optional)
 1 tablespoon grated peeled gingerroot or 1 teaspoon ground ginger
 ½ teaspoon ground turmeric
 ½ teaspoon salt
 1 medium garlic clove, minced
 2 tablespoons chopped fresh cilantro or parsley

In a large, heavy saucepan, bring the water and lentils to a boil over medium-high heat. Reduce the heat and simmer, partially covered, for 45 to 50 minutes, or until tender, skimming off the foam and stirring occasionally.

Meanwhile, heat a medium nonstick skillet over medium-high heat. If using the cumin seeds, cook them for 1 minute, stirring constantly. Watch carefully so they don't burn. Stir in the onion and oil. Stir in the ground cumin if using. Cook for 4 to 5 minutes, or until the onion is lightly browned, stirring occasionally.

Stir in the tomato and chile. Cook for 5 minutes, or until the tomato is reduced to pulp, stirring frequently. Discard the chile.

When the lentils are tender, stir in the onion mixture and the remaining ingredients except the cilantro. Simmer for 10 to 15 minutes.

Just before serving, sprinkle with the cilantro.

COOK'S TIP ON FREEZING GINGERROOT: Many recipes call for just a small amount of fresh gingerroot. To save time in the future, mince or grate the whole root, then divide it into tablespoon-size piles. Place the piles on a baking sheet or plate lined with parchment paper and freeze. Once the gingerroot is frozen, transfer it to an airtight container or resealable plastic freezer bag.

COOK'S TIP ON TURMERIC: Sometimes known as the poor man's saffron because it's more affordable, turmeric adds a beautiful reddish-orange color to foods. It's pungent, so use it sparingly if you just want to enhance the color of your dish.

PER SERVING

Calories 204	Cholesterol 0 mg	DIETARY EXCHANGES:
Total Fat 1.0 g	Sodium 204 mg	2 starch
Saturated Fat 0.0 g	Carbohydrates 37 g	1 vegetable
Trans Fat 0.0 g	Fiber 7 g	1 lean meat
Polyunsaturated Fat 0.5 g	Sugars 6 g	
Monounsaturated Fat 0.5 g	Protein 15 g	

Thai Coconut Curry with Vegetables

Serves 4

This light yet filling stir-fry boasts a hefty helping of vegetables and a spicy coconut-flavored sauce. Lime zest and juice add a final burst of citrus. Serve over steaming brown or jasmine rice if you wish, but this curry is also delicious on its own.

2 teaspoons canola or corn oil
½ medium onion, chopped
2 cups broccoli florets
14 ounces light firm tofu, drained, patted dry, and cut into ½-inch cubes
2 medium carrots, thinly sliced
1 cup canned baby corn, rinsed and drained
1 cup fat-free, low-sodium vegetable broth
⅔ cup lite coconut milk
⅓ cup fat-free evaporated milk
2 teaspoons Thai red curry paste (lowest sodium available)
½ teaspoon coconut extract
2 tablespoons cornstarch
3 tablespoons water
2 teaspoons grated lime zest
1 tablespoon fresh lime juice

In a large nonstick skillet, heat the oil over medium-high heat, swirling to coat the bottom. Cook the onion for 1 to 2 minutes, or until almost soft, stirring frequently.

Stir in the broccoli, tofu, carrots, and corn. Cook for 2 to 3 minutes, or until the broccoli and carrots are tender-crisp, stirring frequently.

Stir in the broth, coconut milk, evaporated milk, curry paste, and coconut extract. Reduce the heat and simmer, covered, for 2 to 3 minutes, or until the vegetables are tender.

Put the cornstarch in a small bowl. Add the water, whisking to dissolve. Stir into the curry. Increase the heat to medium high. Cook for 1 to 2 minutes, or until thickened, stirring occasionally.

Stir in the lime zest and juice.

COOK'S TIP ON CURRY PASTE: A richly flavored blend of dried chiles, pepper, coriander, cumin, lemongrass, galanga (peppery Thai ginger), lime, garlic, and shrimp paste, Thai red curry paste is sold in many supermarkets and in Asian markets.

PER SERVING

Calories 178	Cholesterol 1 mg	DIETARY EXCHANGES:
Total Fat 5.5 g	Sodium 372 mg	1 starch
Saturated Fat 1.5 g	Carbohydrates 22 g	2 vegetable
Trans Fat 0.0 g	Fiber 6 g	1 lean meat
Polyunsaturated Fat 1.0 g	Sugars 7 g	
Monounsaturated Fat 1.5 g	Protein 11 g	

Rosemary-Artichoke Frittata

Serves 4

This Italian omelet bursts with flavor from mushrooms, artichoke hearts, and plenty of herbs. Sweet tomatoes and creamy mozzarella add the crowning touch just before the frittata is broiled to toasty perfection. For a bit of a decadent accompaniment for a special occasion, try Mango Brûlée with Pine Nuts (page 310), which can go under the broiler while the frittata rests.

> Cooking spray
> 4 ounces button mushrooms, sliced
> 9 ounces frozen artichoke hearts, thawed, drained, and coarsely chopped
> 1 cup egg substitute
> ¼ cup fat-free milk
> ¼ cup finely chopped green onions
> ¼ cup finely chopped fresh parsley
> ½ teaspoon dried oregano, crumbled, and ¼ teaspoon dried oregano, crumbled, divided use
> ¼ teaspoon dried rosemary, crushed, and ⅛ teaspoon dried rosemary, crushed, divided use
> 3 medium Italian plum (Roma) tomatoes, thinly sliced
> ⅛ teaspoon salt
> ⅔ cup shredded low-fat mozzarella cheese

Lightly spray a large ovenproof skillet with cooking spray. Cook the mushrooms over medium heat for 3 to 4 minutes, or until slightly soft, stirring occasionally.

In a medium bowl, stir together the artichoke hearts, egg substitute, milk, green onions, parsley, ½ teaspoon oregano, and ¼ teaspoon rosemary. Pour over the mushrooms. Reduce the heat to medium low and cook, covered, without stirring for 10 minutes, or until almost set (the frittata doesn't jiggle when gently shaken and appears to be very moist). Remove from the heat.

Meanwhile, preheat the broiler.

Arrange the tomato slices over the frittata. Sprinkle the salt and the remaining ¼ teaspoon oregano and ⅛ teaspoon rosemary over the tomato slices. Sprinkle the mozzarella over all.

Broil 3 or 4 inches from the heat for 2 minutes, or until the mozzarella is just beginning to turn golden. Let stand for about 5 minutes before cutting into wedges.

COOK'S TIP: Because of the generous amount of moisture in the artichokes, it may appear that the frittata is not cooked at the recommended time. After the frittata stands for a few minutes and the mozzarella has melted, however, the liquid will absorb properly.

PER SERVING

Calories 133	Cholesterol 12 mg	DIETARY EXCHANGES:
Total Fat 3.5 g	Sodium 363 mg	2 vegetable
Saturated Fat 2.0 g	Carbohydrates 12 g	1½ lean meat
Trans Fat 0.0 g	Fiber 6 g	
Polyunsaturated Fat 0.0 g	Sugars 4 g	
Monounsaturated Fat 1.0 g	Protein 14 g	

Watercress-Cheese Soufflé

Serves 6

The light and airy soufflé is one of the most famous creations to emerge from French cooking. This entrée version is made with egg whites and egg substitute and gets its richness from fat-free evaporated milk and low-fat Cheddar. Watercress adds a peppery tang, but you can use cilantro or parsley instead.

3 tablespoons light tub margarine
¼ cup all-purpose flour
1 12-ounce can fat-free evaporated milk
1 cup shredded low-fat sharp Cheddar cheese
¼ cup coarsely chopped watercress, cilantro, or parsley
¾ cup egg substitute
6 large egg whites

Preheat the oven to 350°F.

In a small saucepan, melt the margarine over medium heat, swirling to coat the bottom. Stir in the flour. Pour in the milk. Cook for about 10 minutes, or until thickened and bubbly, stirring frequently. Stir in the Cheddar until melted. Stir in the watercress.

Pour the egg substitute into a medium bowl. Slowly pour in the milk mixture, stirring constantly. Let stand for 5 minutes, or until slightly cooled.

In a large stainless steel or glass mixing bowl, using an electric mixer on high speed, beat the egg whites until stiff peaks form (the peaks don't fall when the beaters are lifted). Using a rubber spatula, gently fold about 2 cups of the egg whites into the egg substitute mixture.

Gradually pour the egg substitute mixture over the remaining egg whites, gently folding to combine. Pour into an ungreased 2-quart soufflé dish. Bake for 50 minutes, or until a knife inserted in the center comes out clean. Serve immediately.

....

COOK'S TIP: Don't use fat-free cheese in this soufflé. It won't melt satisfactorily when it's added to the thickened sauce.

....

COOK'S TIP ON EGG WHITES: Eggs will separate more easily when they're chilled, because the yolk is firmer and less likely to break. To get the best results when beating them, let the separated egg whites come to room temperature and put them in a stainless steel bowl.

PER SERVING

Calories 154	Cholesterol 7 mg	DIETARY EXCHANGES:
Total Fat 4.0 g	Sodium 352 mg	½ starch
Saturated Fat 1.0 g	Carbohydrates 12 g	½ fat-free milk
Trans Fat 0.0 g	Fiber 0 g	1½ lean meat
Polyunsaturated Fat 0.5 g	Sugars 8 g	
Monounsaturated Fat 1.5 g	Protein 17 g	

Edamame Stir-Fry

Serves 4

This speedy stir-fry combines protein-rich edamame with yellow summer squash, tender corn, sweet red bell pepper, and spicy green chiles. Sliced red cabbage adds a crunchy finish.

- 4 cups fat-free, low-sodium vegetable broth or water
- 2 cups frozen edamame
  Cooking spray
- 4 medium garlic cloves, minced
- 2 medium yellow summer squash, diced
- 1 large onion, diced
- 1 medium red bell pepper, diced
- 1 cup frozen whole-kernel corn
- 1 4-ounce can diced green chiles, drained
- 3 tablespoons fresh lemon juice
- 1½ teaspoons ground coriander
- ½ teaspoon ground ginger
- ¼ teaspoon salt
- ⅛ teaspoon pepper
- ¼ medium head red cabbage, thinly sliced

In a large saucepan, stir together the broth and edamame. Bring to a boil over high heat. Reduce the heat and simmer, partially covered, for 6 to 7 minutes, or until the edamame are tender. Drain well in a colander.

Lightly spray a medium skillet with cooking spray. Cook the garlic over medium-low heat for 30 seconds, stirring frequently. Stir in the squash, onion, bell pepper, and corn. Cook for 5 to 7 minutes, or until the vegetables are tender-crisp, stirring frequently.

Stir in the edamame and the remaining ingredients except the cabbage. Cook for 1 to 2 minutes, or until heated through, stirring occasionally.

Just before serving, garnish the stir-fry with the cabbage.

PER SERVING

Calories 226	Cholesterol 0 mg	DIETARY EXCHANGES:
Total Fat 6.0 g	Sodium 272 mg	1 starch
Saturated Fat 1.0 g	Carbohydrates 32 g	3 vegetable
Trans Fat 0.0 g	Fiber 11 g	1 lean meat
Polyunsaturated Fat 3.0 g	Sugars 11 g	½ fat
Monounsaturated Fat 1.0 g	Protein 14 g	

Mediterranean Strata

Serves 6

Although some stratas are layered, ours is simplified and cooked all together, like a savory bread pudding packed with garden vegetables. Pair this with a simple salad for an easy summertime meal.

Cooking spray
1 tablespoon olive oil
2 medium garlic cloves, minced
3 small zucchini (about 12 ounces total), diced
2 medium red bell peppers, thinly sliced
6 slices light whole-grain bread, cubed (lowest sodium available)
½ cup loosely packed fresh basil, coarsely chopped
½ cup cherry tomatoes, halved
1½ cups fat-free, low-sodium vegetable broth
1½ cups egg substitute
¼ cup plus 2 tablespoons shredded or grated Asiago or Parmesan cheese

Preheat the oven to 350°F. Lightly spray a 13 x 9 x 2-inch baking dish with cooking spray.

In a large skillet, heat the oil over medium-high heat, swirling to coat the bottom. Cook the garlic for 10 seconds, stirring constantly. Watch carefully so it doesn't burn. Stir in the zucchini and bell pepper. Cook for 5 to 6 minutes, or until tender-crisp. Transfer to the baking dish. Gently stir in the bread, basil, and tomatoes, spreading evenly.

In a medium bowl, whisk together the broth, egg substitute, and Asiago. Pour over the zucchini mixture. (The strata can be covered and refrigerated for up to 8 hours before baking if desired.)

Bake for 50 to 55 minutes, or until the center is set (the strata doesn't jiggle when gently shaken). (If refrigerated, uncover the strata before placing in a cold oven and baking at 350°F for 1 hour to 1 hour 5 minutes.) Let cool slightly before slicing.

PER SERVING

Calories 141	Cholesterol 4 mg	DIETARY EXCHANGES:
Total Fat 4.5 g	Sodium 339 mg	½ starch
Saturated Fat 1.5 g	Carbohydrates 16 g	1 vegetable
Trans Fat 0.0 g	Fiber 5 g	1 lean meat
Polyunsaturated Fat 0.5 g	Sugars 6 g	
Monounsaturated Fat 2.0 g	Protein 12 g	

Vegetables and Side Dishes

BEETS IN ORANGE SAUCE 248

ASPARAGUS WITH DILL AND PINE NUTS 250

SWEET-AND-SOUR BROCCOLI AND RED BELL PEPPER 251

ROASTED BRUSSELS SPROUTS 252

STIR-FRIED CABBAGE WITH NOODLES 253

CARROT AND BARLEY PILAF 254

APPLE-LEMON CARROTS 255

CAULIFLOWER AU GRATIN 256

TINY CHIVE DUMPLINGS 258

INDIVIDUAL CORN PUDDINGS 259

SWEET-TART GREEN BEANS 260

SAUTÉED GREENS AND CABBAGE 261

TWICE-BAKED POTATOES AND HERBS 262

SWEET POTATOES IN CREAMY CINNAMON SAUCE 263

RED AND GREEN PILAF 264

GOLDEN RICE 265

PRALINE BUTTERNUT SQUASH 266

WILTED SPINACH 268

OVEN-FRIED GREEN TOMATOES WITH POPPY SEEDS 269

STOVETOP SCALLOPED TOMATOES 270

STUFFED ZUCCHINI 271

TRIPLE VEGETABLE BAKE 272

RATATOUILLE 274

VEGETABLE PANCAKES 275

Beets in Orange Sauce

Serves 6

Fresh orange sauce accentuates the rich sweetness of beets. For an even prettier dish, use a mixture of red and golden beets.

2 quarts water
2 pounds beets, stems trimmed to about 1 to 2 inches

SAUCE

1 tablespoon sugar
1 tablespoon cornstarch
1/16 teaspoon salt
2 teaspoons grated orange zest, or to taste
2/3 cup fresh orange juice
1 teaspoon light tub margarine
. . . .
1 medium orange, peeled and divided into sections (optional)

In a large saucepan, bring the water to a boil over high heat. Add the beets. Reduce the heat and simmer, covered, for 40 to 50 minutes, or until tender. Drain well in a colander. Set aside until cool enough to handle.

Meanwhile, in a small saucepan, stir together the sugar, cornstarch, salt, and orange zest. Slowly pour in the orange juice, stirring until smooth. Cook over medium heat for 5 to 8 minutes, or until thickened, stirring constantly.

Add the margarine, stirring until melted.

When the beets have cooled, peel them, discarding the stems. Cut the beets into wedges. Transfer to a serving dish.

Pour the sauce over the beets. Garnish with the orange sections.

COOK'S TIP: You can substitute two 15-ounce cans of no-salt-added whole beets for the fresh beets. Heat them over medium heat, then drain them well before cutting them into wedges and pouring the sauce on top.

COOK'S TIP ON FRESH BEETS: Peel beets under running water to prevent the beet juice from staining your hands. When you're using fresh beets, you shouldn't discard the greens. They're similar to chard. Slice them into thin strips and toss them into a leafy green salad to add color and flavor.

PER SERVING

Calories 94	Cholesterol 0 mg	DIETARY EXCHANGES:
Total Fat 0.5 g	Sodium 147 mg	3 vegetable
Saturated Fat 0.0 g	Carbohydrates 21 g	½ other carbohydrate
Trans Fat 0.0 g	Fiber 4 g	
Polyunsaturated Fat 0.0 g	Sugars 15 g	
Monounsaturated Fat 0.0 g	Protein 3 g	

Asparagus with Dill and Pine Nuts

Serves 4

Take advantage of fresh asparagus during its peak season, February through June, by preparing this tasty side dish. Try it with Tilapia Piccata (page 126) or Broiled Salmon with Olive Pesto (page 122).

1 teaspoon olive oil
2 medium shallots, finely chopped
1 pound asparagus spears, trimmed
2 tablespoons shredded or grated Parmesan cheese
1 tablespoon chopped fresh dillweed or 1 teaspoon dried dillweed, crumbled
1 teaspoon grated lemon zest
⅛ teaspoon pepper
2 tablespoons pine nuts, dry-roasted

In a large nonstick skillet, heat the oil over medium heat, swirling to coat the bottom. Cook the shallots for 1 to 2 minutes, or until tender-crisp, stirring frequently.

Add the asparagus. Cook for 3 to 4 minutes, or until tender-crisp, stirring occasionally.

Stir in the remaining ingredients except the pine nuts. Cook for 1 minute, or until the Parmesan is melted, stirring occasionally.

Sprinkle with the pine nuts.

PER SERVING

Calories 68	Cholesterol 2 mg	DIETARY EXCHANGES:
Total Fat 4.0 g	Sodium 46 mg	1 vegetable
Saturated Fat 1.0 g	Carbohydrates 6 g	1 fat
Trans Fat 0.0 g	Fiber 3 g	
Polyunsaturated Fat 1.0 g	Sugars 3 g	
Monounsaturated Fat 2.0 g	Protein 5 g	

Sweet-and-Sour Broccoli and Red Bell Pepper

Serves 6

Take this innovative, Asian-inspired side dish along on your next picnic. It doesn't need space in the cooler and, thanks to the tangy dressing, it will perk up simple grilled chicken and meats.

> 1 **pound broccoli florets**
> 1 **medium red bell pepper, cut into thin strips**
> ½ **cup plain rice vinegar**
> 3 **tablespoons light brown sugar**
> 1 **medium green onion (green part only), thinly sliced**
> 1 **tablespoon plus 1 teaspoon soy sauce (lowest sodium available)**
> 1 **tablespoon grated peeled gingerroot**
> 1 **tablespoon toasted sesame oil**
> 2 **medium garlic cloves, minced**
> 2 **tablespoons sliced almonds, dry-roasted**

In a large saucepan, steam the broccoli and bell pepper for 5 to 7 minutes, or until tender-crisp. Plunge into cold water to stop the cooking process. Drain well in a colander. Dry on paper towels. Transfer to a medium serving bowl.

In a small bowl, whisk together the remaining ingredients except the almonds. Pour over the broccoli mixture. Toss gently to coat. Cover and refrigerate for at least 1 hour so the flavors blend.

Shortly before serving, bring to room temperature. Sprinkle with the almonds.

PER SERVING

Calories 95	Cholesterol 0 mg	DIETARY EXCHANGES:
Total Fat 3.5 g	Sodium 116 mg	1 vegetable
Saturated Fat 0.5 g	Carbohydrates 15 g	½ other carbohydrate
Trans Fat 0.0 g	Fiber 3 g	1 fat
Polyunsaturated Fat 1.5 g	Sugars 10 g	
Monounsaturated Fat 1.5 g	Protein 3 g	

Roasted Brussels Sprouts

Serves 4

Roasting brings out the natural sweetness of brussels sprouts, while balsamic vinegar enhances their nutty flavor and Dijon adds a mild tang that's tempered by just a hint of brown sugar. Once you try these, you'll be hooked.

Cooking spray
8 ounces medium brussels sprouts, trimmed and halved lengthwise

DRESSING

1 tablespoon balsamic vinegar
1 tablespoon Dijon mustard (lowest sodium available)
2 teaspoons olive oil (extra virgin preferred)
1 medium garlic clove, minced
½ teaspoon light brown sugar
¼ teaspoon pepper

Preheat the oven to 400°F. Lightly spray a 13 x 9 x 2-inch glass baking dish with cooking spray.

Arrange the brussels sprouts in a single layer in the baking dish. Lightly spray with cooking spray.

Roast for 20 to 25 minutes, or until tender when pierced with the tip of a sharp knife, stirring once or twice.

Meanwhile, in a large serving bowl, whisk together the dressing ingredients.

Add the sprouts to the dressing, stirring to coat. Serve warm or cover and refrigerate for up to three days to serve cold.

PER SERVING		
Calories 56	Cholesterol 0 mg	DIETARY EXCHANGES:
Total Fat 2.5 g	Sodium 92 mg	1 vegetable
Saturated Fat 0.5 g	Carbohydrates 7 g	½ fat
Trans Fat 0.0 g	Fiber 2 g	
Polyunsaturated Fat 0.5 g	Sugars 3 g	
Monounsaturated Fat 1.5 g	Protein 2 g	

Stir-Fried Cabbage with Noodles

Serves 5

Cabbage and pasta may seem to be unlikely partners, but they work well together in this traditional Eastern European dish. Earthy, slightly peppery caraway seeds, familiar to fans of rye bread, add character to the cabbage.

1 cup dried no-yolk noodles
1 tablespoon light tub margarine
3 cups finely chopped green cabbage
¾ teaspoon caraway seeds
½ teaspoon onion powder

Prepare the noodles using the package directions, omitting the salt. Drain well in a colander.

Meanwhile, in a large skillet, melt the margarine over medium heat, swirling to coat the bottom. Cook the cabbage for 5 to 8 minutes, or until tender-crisp, stirring frequently.

Stir in the noodles, caraway seeds, and onion powder.

PER SERVING

Calories 54	Cholesterol 0 mg	DIETARY EXCHANGES:
Total Fat 1.0 g	Sodium 30 mg	½ starch
Saturated Fat 0.0 g	Carbohydrates 10 g	
Trans Fat 0.0 g	Fiber 2 g	
Polyunsaturated Fat 0.0 g	Sugars 2 g	
Monounsaturated Fat 0.5 g	Protein 2 g	

Carrot and Barley Pilaf

Serves 4

The convenience, flavor, and texture of quick-cooking barley will make you want to prepare this whole-grain side dish often instead of reaching for the usual go-to, rice. It pairs nicely with roasted pork tenderloin, such as Pork with Savory Sauce (page 203), or grilled salmon, such as Mediterranean Grilled Salmon (page 123).

1⅓ cups fat-free, low-sodium chicken broth
⅔ cup uncooked quick-cooking barley
1 teaspoon olive oil
2 medium carrots, shredded
2 medium green onions, thinly sliced
2 tablespoons chopped pecans, dry-roasted
½ teaspoon ground cumin
⅛ teaspoon salt
⅛ teaspoon pepper

In a medium saucepan, bring the broth to a boil over medium-high heat. Stir in the barley. Reduce the heat and simmer, covered, for 10 to 12 minutes, or until the barley is tender and almost all the liquid is absorbed. Remove from the heat. Let stand, covered, for 5 minutes. Fluff with a fork.

Meanwhile, in a medium skillet, heat the oil over medium-high heat, swirling to coat the bottom. Stir in the remaining ingredients. Cook for 1 to 2 minutes, or until the carrots are tender-crisp. Stir into the cooked barley.

PER SERVING

Calories 175	Cholesterol 0 mg	DIETARY EXCHANGES:
Total Fat 4.0 g	Sodium 124 mg	1½ starch
Saturated Fat 0.5 g	Carbohydrates 31 g	1 vegetable
Trans Fat 0.0 g	Fiber 7 g	½ fat
Polyunsaturated Fat 1.0 g	Sugars 3 g	
Monounsaturated Fat 2.5 g	Protein 5 g	

Apple-Lemon Carrots

Serves 6

Tired of plain carrots? Give them a fruity twist with a touch of apple and lemon juice. This sweet side pairs well with Crispy Oven-Fried Chicken (page 144) or Ham and Rice Croquettes (page 204).

1 pound carrots, grated
2 tablespoons frozen 100% apple juice concentrate, thawed
1 tablespoon fresh lemon juice
1 teaspoon light tub margarine
1 teaspoon poppy seeds

In a medium nonstick skillet, stir together the carrots, apple juice concentrate, and lemon juice. Cook over medium-high heat for 3 minutes, or until the carrots are tender, stirring constantly.

Add the margarine, stirring to coat the carrots. Just before serving, sprinkle with the poppy seeds.

PER SERVING

Calories 46	Cholesterol 0 mg	DIETARY EXCHANGES:
Total Fat 0.5 g	Sodium 59 mg	2 vegetable
Saturated Fat 0.0 g	Carbohydrates 10 g	
Trans Fat 0.0 g	Fiber 2 g	
Polyunsaturated Fat 0.5 g	Sugars 6 g	
Monounsaturated Fat 0.0 g	Protein 1 g	

Cauliflower au Gratin

Serves 8

Just as satisfying as classic cauliflower with cheese sauce but updated to be heart-healthy, this soothing side dish has everything you expect: mild cauliflower, creamy texture, and crisp topping. Try it with Meat Loaf with Apricot Glaze (page 192).

1   medium head of cauliflower (about 1½ pounds), cut into florets, or 20 ounces frozen cauliflower florets
½   teaspoon salt-free all-purpose seasoning
½   cup fat-free milk
½   cup fat-free, low-sodium chicken broth
1½ tablespoons all-purpose flour
⅛   teaspoon ground nutmeg
½   cup shredded low-fat sharp Cheddar cheese
2   tablespoons whole-wheat panko (Japanese-style bread crumbs)
2   tablespoons shredded or grated Parmesan cheese

If using fresh cauliflower, steam it for 8 to 10 minutes, or until tender, in a large saucepan. If using frozen cauliflower, prepare using the package directions. Drain well in a colander if needed. Sprinkle the cooked cauliflower with the seasoning blend. Transfer to an 8-inch square nonstick baking dish.

Preheat the oven to 350°F.

In a small saucepan, whisk together the milk, broth, flour, and nutmeg. Bring to a simmer over medium-high heat, whisking constantly to prevent scorching. Adjusting the heat if necessary, simmer for 2 to 3 minutes, or until thickened, whisking constantly. Reduce the heat to medium low.

Stir in the Cheddar. Cook for 1 minute, or until melted, whisking occasionally. Pour over the cauliflower, stirring to coat.

In a small bowl, stir together the panko and Parmesan. Sprinkle over the cauliflower mixture.

Bake for 20 minutes, or until golden brown on top.

COOK'S TIP ON PANKO: Panko is coarser, lighter, and usually lower in sodium than regular bread crumbs. Though these products are interchangeable in almost any recipe, panko produces a crisper crust when baked. To find panko, look for it in the Asian section of your supermarket or the aisle where the traditional bread crumbs are found. Be sure to buy plain or unseasoned varieties, which are much lower in sodium.

PER SERVING

Calories 50	Cholesterol 3 mg	DIETARY EXCHANGES:
Total Fat 1.0 g	Sodium 98 mg	1 vegetable
Saturated Fat 0.5 g	Carbohydrates 6 g	½ lean meat
Trans Fat 0.0 g	Fiber 2 g	
Polyunsaturated Fat 0.0 g	Sugars 2 g	
Monounsaturated Fat 0.5 g	Protein 5 g	

Tiny Chive Dumplings

Serves 4

These small, puffy morsels are inspired by *spaetzle,* a cross between a noodle and a dumpling. *Spaetzle* traditionally accompany goulash and all types of roasts, such as Beef Tenderloin Roast (page 180).

- 1 cup all-purpose flour
- ⅛ teaspoon salt
- ⅛ teaspoon pepper
- ⅓ cup fat-free milk
- ¼ cup egg substitute
- 2 tablespoons finely chopped chives

Fill a Dutch oven three-quarters full with water. Bring to a boil over high heat.

Meanwhile, in a medium mixing bowl, stir together the flour, salt, and pepper. Make a well in the center.

In a small bowl, whisk together the milk and egg substitute. Pour into the well in the flour mixture. Add the chives, stirring until well combined but no flour is visible.

Hold a colander with large holes over the boiling water. Pour the batter into the colander. Using a long-handled spoon, press the batter through the holes in the colander so streams of batter fall into the water. Cook for 5 minutes, stirring occasionally. Drain well in a clean colander.

....

cook's tip: You can even toss these dumplings with a small amount of olive oil if you're serving them with a main dish that doesn't have a sauce or broth.

....

PER SERVING

Calories 129	Cholesterol 0 mg	DIETARY EXCHANGES:
Total Fat 0.5 g	Sodium 113 mg	1½ starch
Saturated Fat 0.0 g	Carbohydrates 25 g	
Trans Fat 0.0 g	Fiber 1 g	
Polyunsaturated Fat 0.0 g	Sugars 1 g	
Monounsaturated Fat 0.0 g	Protein 6 g	

Individual Corn Puddings

Serves 4

Creamy corn pudding is usually loaded with saturated fat. This version cuts the fat but none of the flavor. Use fresh corn during the summer, when it's at its peak, but frozen corn works just as well the rest of the year.

Cooking spray
1 cup fat-free milk
¼ cup egg substitute
1 tablespoon olive oil
¼ teaspoon pepper
⅓ cup all-purpose flour
1 cup corn kernels, cut from 1 large or 2 small ears of corn, husks and silk discarded, or 1 cup frozen whole-kernel corn, thawed

Preheat the oven to 350°F. Lightly spray four 8-ounce custard cups with cooking spray. Put on a baking sheet.

In a medium bowl, whisk together the milk, egg substitute, oil, and pepper.

Add the flour, whisking just until combined but no flour is visible. The mixture will be lumpy.

Stir in the corn. Spoon into the custard cups.

Bake for 35 to 40 minutes, or until the center is set (the pudding doesn't jiggle when gently shaken) or a wooden toothpick inserted in the center comes out clean. The corn pudding will rise like a soufflé, then fall quickly when removed from the oven.

PER SERVING

Calories 127	Cholesterol 1 mg	DIETARY EXCHANGES:
Total Fat 4.0 g	Sodium 63 mg	1 starch
Saturated Fat 0.5 g	Carbohydrates 18 g	½ lean meat
Trans Fat 0.0 g	Fiber 1 g	½ fat
Polyunsaturated Fat 0.5 g	Sugars 6 g	
Monounsaturated Fat 2.5 g	Protein 6 g	

Sweet-Tart Green Beans

Serves 4

These lemony green beans have just a touch of sweetness. They pair well with nearly any entrée, but their light flavor is especially good with Slow-Cooker Pepper Steak (page 190) or Poached Halibut in Asian Broth (page 118).

1   pound green beans, trimmed and cut into 1-inch pieces, or 10 ounces frozen cut green beans, thawed
1   teaspoon light tub margarine
½   teaspoon all-purpose flour
1   tablespoon sugar
1   tablespoon water
1   tablespoon fresh lemon juice
¼   teaspoon dill seeds (optional)
⅛   teaspoon paprika

In a large saucepan, steam the green beans for 3 to 5 minutes, or until tender. Drain well in a colander.

Meanwhile, in a medium skillet, melt the margarine over medium heat, swirling to coat the bottom. Stir in the flour. Cook for 2 to 3 minutes, or until lightly browned, stirring frequently. Stir in the remaining ingredients. Reduce the heat to low and cook for 2 to 3 minutes, or until the sauce is thickened, stirring occasionally.

Transfer the green beans to a medium serving bowl. Pour the sauce over the green beans, stirring to combine. Serve immediately.

PER SERVING

Calories 53	Cholesterol 0 mg	DIETARY EXCHANGES:
Total Fat 0.5 g	Sodium 15 mg	2 vegetable
Saturated Fat 0.0 g	Carbohydrates 12 g	
Trans Fat 0.0 g	Fiber 3 g	
Polyunsaturated Fat 0.0 g	Sugars 7 g	
Monounsaturated Fat 0.0 g	Protein 2 g	

Sautéed Greens and Cabbage

Serves 6

Cabbage and rice vinegar enhance the flavor of the greens used in this simple dish. Try it with southern favorites such as Crisp Catfish with Creole Sauce (page 112) or Crispy Oven-Fried Chicken (page 144).

3 quarts water
1 bunch of collard greens, kale, turnip greens, or spinach (12 to 16 ounces), stems discarded, leaves finely chopped
⅓ medium head of green cabbage, coarsely shredded (2½ to 3 cups)
    Olive oil cooking spray
1 teaspoon olive oil
1 medium onion, quartered and sliced
1 medium garlic clove, minced
2 teaspoons plain rice vinegar or white wine vinegar
¼ teaspoon salt
    Red hot-pepper sauce to taste

In a large saucepan or Dutch oven, bring the water to a boil over high heat. Stir in the greens. Return to a boil. Cook for 3 to 4 minutes, or until tender-crisp. Using a large slotted spoon, transfer the greens to a colander, leaving the water in the pan. Drain the greens and leave them in the colander.

Return the water to a boil, still over high heat. Stir in the cabbage. Cook for 1 minute. Drain in the colander with the greens.

Reduce the heat to medium low. Lightly spray a large skillet with cooking spray. Pour in the oil, swirling to coat the bottom. Cook the onion and garlic for 2 to 3 minutes, or until slightly soft, stirring occasionally.

Stir in the greens and cabbage. Cook for 2 to 3 minutes, or until heated through, stirring occasionally.

Stir in the vinegar, salt, and hot-pepper sauce.

PER SERVING

Calories 45	Cholesterol 0 mg	DIETARY EXCHANGES:
Total Fat 1.0 g	Sodium 172 mg	2 vegetable
Saturated Fat 0.0 g	Carbohydrates 8 g	
Trans Fat 0.0 g	Fiber 4 g	
Polyunsaturated Fat 0.0 g	Sugars 4 g	
Monounsaturated Fat 0.5 g	Protein 2 g	

Twice-Baked Potatoes and Herbs

Serves 4

Varying the fresh herbs gives you lots of options for these creamy, cheesy potatoes. A delectable change from plain baked potatoes, they pair especially well with simple roasted poultry or meats.

- **4 medium baking potatoes (russets preferred), pierced with a fork in several places**
- **⅓ cup fat-free sour cream or fat-free plain Greek yogurt**
- **2 tablespoons chopped fresh herbs, such as basil, chives, thyme, marjoram, oregano, parsley, or any combination**
- **2 tablespoons shredded or grated Parmesan cheese**
- **1 to 2 tablespoons fat-free milk (as needed)**
- **¼ cup shredded low-fat mozzarella cheese**

Preheat the oven to 425°F. Put the potatoes on a baking sheet.

Bake for 40 minutes to 1 hour, or until tender. Transfer the potatoes to a cooling rack. Let cool.

Cut a thin lengthwise slice from the top of each potato. Using a spoon, carefully scoop out all the pulp from those slices and discard the skins. Scoop out most of the pulp from each potato, leaving a ¼-inch border of the shell all the way around. Transfer the pulp to a large mixing bowl.

Using an electric mixer on low speed or a potato masher, beat or mash the potato pulp. Stir in the sour cream, herbs, and Parmesan. Beat or mash until smooth. Stir in enough milk to reach the desired consistency. Spoon into the shells. Place in a medium shallow baking dish. Sprinkle the mozzarella over the potatoes.

Bake for 15 to 20 minutes, or until lightly browned.

....

COOK'S TIP ON LEFTOVER FRESH HERBS: Small amounts of fresh herbs, such as basil, parsley, cilantro, or a mixture, are needed ingredients for healthy and flavorful dips and salad dressings, such as Fresh Basil and Kalamata Hummus (page 34) and Creamy Herb Dressing (page 98).

....

PER SERVING
....

Calories 159	Cholesterol 8 mg	DIETARY EXCHANGES:
Total Fat 1.5 g	Sodium 119 mg	2 starch
Saturated Fat 0.5 g	Carbohydrates 27 g	½ lean meat
Trans Fat 0.0 g	Fiber 2 g	
Polyunsaturated Fat 0.0 g	Sugars 3 g	
Monounsaturated Fat 0.5 g	**Protein 7 g**	

Sweet Potatoes in Creamy Cinnamon Sauce

Serves 6

The aroma of warm spices fills the air as this dish bakes. It's perfect for the holiday season or anytime you want a boost from vitamin-rich sweet potatoes. Serve with Beef Tenderloin Roast (page 180) and Roasted Brussels Sprouts (page 252), which cook at the same temperature.

- 1 **pound sweet potatoes (about 2 large), peeled and cut crosswise into ¼-inch slices**
- ½ **cup fat-free half-and-half**
- 2 **tablespoons light brown sugar**
- 1 **teaspoon grated orange zest**
- ½ **teaspoon ground cinnamon**
- ¼ **teaspoon ground nutmeg**
- 1 **tablespoon light tub margarine**

Preheat the oven to 400°F.

Arrange the sweet potato slices in even layers in an 8-inch round or square nonstick baking pan.

In a small bowl, whisk together the remaining ingredients except the margarine. Pour over the sweet potatoes.

Dot with the margarine.

Bake for 35 to 40 minutes, or until the sweet potatoes are tender, stirring once halfway through.

PER SERVING

Calories 97	Cholesterol 0 mg	DIETARY EXCHANGES:
Total Fat 1.0 g	Sodium 77 mg	1 starch
Saturated Fat 0.0 g	Carbohydrates 21 g	½ other carbohydrate
Trans Fat 0.0 g	Fiber 3 g	
Polyunsaturated Fat 0.0 g	Sugars 10 g	
Monounsaturated Fat 0.5 g	Protein 3 g	

Red and Green Pilaf

Serves 4

Jazz up ordinary brown rice with fresh veggies and just enough cayenne so this side dish gets noticed.

Cooking spray
½ large onion, chopped
⅓ medium green bell pepper, chopped
⅓ medium red bell pepper, chopped
½ cup uncooked brown rice
2 medium garlic cloves, minced
1½ cups fat-free, low-sodium chicken broth
⅛ teaspoon salt
⅛ teaspoon cayenne
1 cup sliced fresh or frozen okra, thawed if frozen, or
⅔ cup fresh or frozen green peas, thawed if frozen
1 medium Italian plum (Roma) tomato, seeds discarded, chopped

Lightly spray a medium saucepan with cooking spray. Cook the onion and bell peppers over medium-high heat for 5 minutes, or until soft, stirring occasionally.

Stir in the rice and garlic. Cook for 1 minute.

Stir in the broth, salt, and cayenne. Increase the heat to high and bring to a boil. Reduce the heat and simmer, covered, for 30 minutes.

Stir in the okra. Cook, covered, for 5 to 10 minutes, or until the rice is tender and the liquid is absorbed.

Stir in the tomato. Let stand for 5 minutes.

PER SERVING

Calories 118	Cholesterol 0 mg	DIETARY EXCHANGES:
Total Fat 1.0 g	Sodium 103 mg	1½ starch
Saturated Fat 0.0 g	Carbohydrates 24 g	1 vegetable
Trans Fat 0.0 g	Fiber 3 g	
Polyunsaturated Fat 0.5 g	Sugars 3 g	
Monounsaturated Fat 0.5 g	Protein 4 g	

Golden Rice

Serves 6

Turmeric or saffron gives this rice dish its bright yellow hue while also adding an exotic flavor when combined with cinnamon and almonds. An impeccable partner for Middle Eastern, Greek, or Indian cuisine, this rice can also add intrigue to a simple roasted or broiled entrée.

1 cup fat-free, low-sodium chicken broth
1 cup water
1 cup uncooked brown basmati or other long-grain rice
1 cinnamon stick (about 3 inches long)
1 medium dried bay leaf
¼ teaspoon salt
¼ teaspoon ground turmeric or saffron
2 tablespoons slivered almonds, dry-roasted

In a medium saucepan, bring the broth and water to a boil over medium-high heat. Stir in the rice, cinnamon stick, bay leaf, and salt. Reduce the heat and simmer, covered, for 20 minutes.

Using a fork, gently stir in the turmeric. Cook, covered, over low heat for 10 minutes, or until the rice is tender and the liquid is absorbed. Discard the cinnamon stick and bay leaf.

Just before serving, sprinkle with the almonds.

....

COOK'S TIP ON BASMATI RICE: In Hindi, *basmati* means "fragrant," which aptly describes the aroma of this long-grain rice. Basmati rice is aged after harvest, which lessens its moisture content and intensifies its distinctive nutlike flavor. Several varieties, such as Texmati and Kasmati, are now grown in the United States. Store the rice in a cool, dry area in a sealed container.

....

PER SERVING

Calories 130	Cholesterol 0 mg	DIETARY EXCHANGES:
Total Fat 2.0 g	Sodium 113 mg	1½ starch
Saturated Fat 0.5 g	Carbohydrates 24 g	
Trans Fat 0.0 g	Fiber 2 g	
Polyunsaturated Fat 0.5 g	Sugars 1 g	
Monounsaturated Fat 1.0 g	Protein 4 g	

Praline Butternut Squash

Serves 8

Pureed butternut squash topped with maple-flavored fruit and pecans—this is a perfect dish for fall and winter entertaining, especially during the holidays.

1   **2- to 2½-pound butternut squash, halved lengthwise, seeds and strings discarded**

1   **cup water**

1   **15.25-ounce can pineapple chunks in their own juice, drained**

½   **cup dried fruit, such as apricots, peaches, apples, or any combination, diced**

2   **tablespoons chopped pecans, dry-roasted**

2   **tablespoons pure maple syrup**

1   **tablespoon dark brown sugar**

1   **teaspoon grated lemon zest**

Preheat the oven to 350°F.

Put the squash with the cut sides down in a shallow baking dish. Pour the water around the squash.

Bake for 45 to 50 minutes, or until the squash is tender. Transfer to a cooling rack. Let cool for at least 15 minutes.

Using a spoon, scoop out the squash pulp, discarding the skin. In a food processor, process the pulp for 1 minute, or until smooth. (You can use a potato masher if you prefer.) Spoon into a 1-quart glass casserole dish.

In a medium bowl, stir together the remaining ingredients. Spoon over the squash.

Bake for 30 minutes, or until heated through.

....

COOK'S TIP ON CUTTING DRIED FRUIT: To prevent your scissors or knife from becoming sticky when you snip or chop dried fruit, lightly spray the utensil with cooking spray or dip it in hot water before using it.

....

COOK'S TIP ON BUTTERNUT SQUASH: Cutting butternut squash is easier if you have the right tools and a little know-how. Here's one method to try: Using a sharp knife, cut a few large slits in the skin. Microwave the squash on 100 percent power (high) for 3 minutes. Remove from the microwave oven. Let stand for 3 to 5 minutes, or until cool enough to handle. Slice off the top and bottom of the squash, then halve the squash lengthwise. The microwaving softens the squash, making it a little easier to cut.

PER SERVING

Calories 130	Cholesterol 0 mg	DIETARY EXCHANGES:
Total Fat 1.5 g	Sodium 21 mg	1 starch
Saturated Fat 0.0 g	Carbohydrates 31 g	1 fruit
Trans Fat 0.0 g	Fiber 4 g	
Polyunsaturated Fat 0.5 g	Sugars 17 g	
Monounsaturated Fat 0.5 g	Protein 2 g	

Wilted Spinach

Serves 4

If you like wilted spinach salad, you'll love this cooked version and its warm sweet-and-sour dressing. You can leave out the chopped egg whites to save time, but they add a nice color contrast to the dish.

> 1　teaspoon olive oil
> 2　medium green onions, thinly sliced
> 2　medium garlic cloves, minced
> 1　pound baby spinach
> 1　tablespoon white wine vinegar
> 1　teaspoon capers, drained
> 1　teaspoon grated lemon zest
> 1　teaspoon light brown sugar
> ⅛　teaspoon pepper
> 2　large hard-boiled egg whites, chopped

In a large nonstick skillet, heat the oil over medium heat, swirling to coat the bottom. Cook the green onions and garlic for 1 to 2 minutes, or until the green onions are tender-crisp, stirring occasionally.

Stir in the spinach. Reduce the heat to medium low and cook, covered, for 3 to 4 minutes, or until the spinach is wilted and soft.

Stir in the remaining ingredients except the egg whites. Cook, covered, for 1 to 2 minutes, or until the mixture is heated through. Transfer to a small serving bowl.

Sprinkle with the egg whites.

....

COOK'S TIP ON HARD-BOILING EGGS: To hard-boil eggs, place them in a small saucepan with a lid. Cover with cold water by 1 to 2 inches. Bring to a full, rolling boil. Remove from the heat. Let the pan stand, covered, for 15 minutes. Plunge the eggs into a bowl of ice water to stop the cooking process. Tap the eggs or roll them on a flat surface to crack the shells. Peel the eggs under cool running water to easily release the white from the shell.

....

PER SERVING

Calories 58	Cholesterol 0 mg	DIETARY EXCHANGES:
Total Fat 1.5 g	Sodium 141 mg	1 vegetable
Saturated Fat 0.0 g	Carbohydrates 7 g	½ lean meat
Trans Fat 0.0 g	Fiber 3 g	
Polyunsaturated Fat 0.5 g	Sugars 2 g	
Monounsaturated Fat 1.0 g	Protein 5 g	

Oven-Fried Green Tomatoes with Poppy Seeds

Serves 6

A typical end-of-summer tradition in the South is to pick the last of the garden tomatoes while they are still green, slice them, coat them with cornmeal, and fry them. This dish captures the same tradition and flavor, but in a healthier way.

Cooking spray
¼ cup egg substitute
2 tablespoons fat-free milk
½ cup cornmeal
¼ cup all-purpose flour
1 teaspoon poppy seeds
¼ teaspoon salt
⅛ teaspoon pepper
1 pound green tomatoes or firm red tomatoes (about 3 medium), cut crosswise into ¼-inch slices

Preheat the oven to 450°F. Lightly spray a baking sheet with cooking spray.

In a small bowl, whisk together the egg substitute and milk. In a pie pan or shallow baking pan, stir together the remaining ingredients except the tomatoes. Put the bowl, pie pan, and baking sheet in a row, assembly-line fashion. Using tongs, dip the tomatoes in the egg substitute mixture, then in the cornmeal mixture, turning to coat at each step and gently shaking off any excess. Using your fingertips, gently press the coating so it adheres to the tomatoes. Arrange the tomatoes in a single layer on the baking sheet.

Bake for 10 minutes. Turn over the tomatoes. Bake for 5 minutes, or until golden brown.

PER SERVING

Calories 86	Cholesterol 0 mg	DIETARY EXCHANGES:
Total Fat 0.5 g	Sodium 130 mg	1 starch
Saturated Fat 0.0 g	Carbohydrates 18 g	1 vegetable
Trans Fat 0.0 g	Fiber 2 g	
Polyunsaturated Fat 0.5 g	Sugars 4 g	
Monounsaturated Fat 0.0 g	Protein 4 g	

Stovetop Scalloped Tomatoes

Serves 4

This twist on the popular casserole-style side dish doesn't require an oven, so it's a perfect way to use fresh summer tomatoes without heating up the kitchen. Serve with Ham and Rice Croquettes (page 204) or with Cajun Red Scallops (page 136).

- 1 slice whole-grain bread (lowest sodium available)
- 1 teaspoon light tub margarine
- 3 medium green or red tomatoes, diced (about 2 cups)
- ¼ cup bell pepper, finely chopped (use green bell pepper with red tomatoes, or red bell pepper with green tomatoes)
- ¼ cup chopped celery
- ¼ cup finely chopped onion (Vidalia, Maui, or Oso Sweet preferred)
- 2 tablespoons water
- 1 tablespoon cornstarch
- 1 tablespoon chopped fresh basil or 1 teaspoon dried basil, crumbled
- 1 teaspoon sugar
- ¼ teaspoon salt

Toast the bread. Spread the margarine over both sides. Cut into 16 cubes. Set aside.

In a medium saucepan, stir together the tomatoes, bell pepper, celery, and onion. Bring to a boil over high heat. Reduce the heat to low. Cook, covered, for 10 minutes, or until the tomatoes and onion are soft and the bell pepper and celery are tender-crisp.

In a small bowl, stir together the remaining ingredients. Stir into the tomato mixture. Increase the heat to medium high and bring to a simmer. Reduce the heat and simmer for 1 to 2 minutes, or until thickened and bubbly, stirring constantly.

Just before serving, garnish with the toast cubes.

PER SERVING

Calories 56	Cholesterol 0 mg	DIETARY EXCHANGES:
Total Fat 1.0 g	Sodium 188 mg	½ starch
Saturated Fat 0.0 g	Carbohydrates 11 g	1 vegetable
Trans Fat 0.0 g	Fiber 2 g	
Polyunsaturated Fat 0.5 g	Sugars 5 g	
Monounsaturated Fat 0.5 g	Protein 2 g	

Stuffed Zucchini

Serves 6

Zucchini is an ancient vegetable that stands alone or serves well as a backdrop for other flavors. In this dish, the hollowed-out squash cradles a savory Mediterranean-inspired stuffing that complements the vegetable's own delicate aroma and flavor. These pair perfectly with the flavors of Chicken Breasts Stuffed with Ricotta and Goat Cheese (page 146). Both recipes also bake at the same oven temperature for the same amount of time!

3 **large zucchini (about 10 ounces each)**
1 **cup plain dry bread crumbs (lowest sodium available)**
3 **large Italian plum (Roma) tomatoes, chopped**
2 **tablespoons fresh lemon juice**
1 **teaspoon dried oregano, crumbled**
¼ **teaspoon pepper**
2 **tablespoons shredded or grated Romano or Parmesan cheese**
⅓ **cup fat-free, low-sodium chicken broth**

Preheat the oven to 350°F.

Halve the zucchini lengthwise. Scoop out the pulp, leaving a ¼-inch border of the shell all the way around. Dice the pulp. Set aside.

In a medium bowl, stir together the zucchini pulp, bread crumbs, tomatoes, lemon juice, oregano, and pepper. Using your hands, squeeze the mixture to moisten thoroughly. Spoon the mixture into the zucchini shells. Sprinkle the Romano over the stuffing. Transfer the stuffed zucchini to a 13 x 9 x 2-inch baking dish. Pour the broth around the zucchini, being careful not to pour it over them.

Bake for 40 minutes, or until a knife inserted in the center goes in easily and the zucchini are tender. Serve hot, warm, or chilled.

PER SERVING

Calories 115	Cholesterol 1 mg	DIETARY EXCHANGES:
Total Fat 2.0 g	Sodium 176 mg	1 starch
Saturated Fat 0.5 g	Carbohydrates 20 g	1 vegetable
Trans Fat 0.0 g	Fiber 3 g	
Polyunsaturated Fat 0.5 g	Sugars 6 g	
Monounsaturated Fat 0.5 g	Protein 6 g	

Triple Vegetable Bake

Serves 6

You'll be hooked after just one bite of this rich, creamy casserole. It cooks at the same temperature as Cumin-Roasted Turkey Breast with Raspberry Sauce (page 174), so you can have your entrée and side dish done at the same time.

Cooking spray

SAUCE

- 1 teaspoon olive oil
- 1 cup finely chopped onion (about 2 medium)
- 8 ounces mushrooms, such as shiitake (stems discarded) or button, quartered
- 6 medium garlic cloves
- ¼ cup white whole-wheat flour
- 1½ cups fat-free milk
- 1 cup fat-free, low-sodium chicken broth
- ⅓ cup dry white wine (regular or nonalcoholic)
- 2 tablespoons finely chopped fresh parsley
- ¼ teaspoon pepper (white preferred)
- ⅛ teaspoon salt
  ·······
- 2 pounds potatoes, peeled and cubed
- 8 ounces broccoli florets

Preheat the oven to 325°F. Lightly spray an 8-inch square baking dish with cooking spray.

In a large nonstick skillet, heat the oil over medium heat, swirling to coat the bottom. Cook the onions, mushrooms, and garlic, covered, for 5 minutes. Increase the heat to medium high. Uncover and cook for 3 to 5 minutes, or until the juices have evaporated, stirring occasionally.

Meanwhile, put the flour in a small bowl. Add the milk, whisking until smooth. Pour into the onion mixture. Whisk in the remaining sauce ingredients. Cook for 3 to 4 minutes, or until thickened, whisking constantly.

Arrange half the potatoes to completely cover the bottom of the baking dish. Pour half the sauce over the potatoes. Repeat with the remaining potatoes and sauce. Bake for 1½ hours.

Meanwhile, in a medium saucepan, steam the broccoli for 5 to 6 minutes, or until tender-crisp. Drain well in a colander. Just before serving, arrange the broccoli in a border around the potatoes.

VARIATION: To turn this side dish into an entrée, combine 1 cup diced, skinless turkey or chicken breast (cooked without salt, all visible fat discarded) and ½ cup lower-sodium, low-fat ham. Place half the mixture on top of each layer of potatoes. Bake as directed.

PER SERVING

Calories 208	Cholesterol 1 mg	DIETARY EXCHANGES:
Total Fat 1.5 g	Sodium 105 mg	2 starch
Saturated Fat 0.0 g	Carbohydrates 40 g	2 vegetable
Trans Fat 0.0 g	Fiber 6 g	
Polyunsaturated Fat 0.5 g	Sugars 7 g	
Monounsaturated Fat 0.5 g	Protein 9 g	

PER SERVING (VARIATION)

Calories 261	Cholesterol 26 mg	DIETARY EXCHANGES:
Total Fat 3.0 g	Sodium 221 mg	2 starch
Saturated Fat 0.5 g	Carbohydrates 40 g	2 vegetable
Trans Fat 0.0 g	Fiber 6 g	1½ lean meat
Polyunsaturated Fat 0.5 g	Sugars 7 g	
Monounsaturated Fat 1.0 g	Protein 18 g	

Ratatouille

Serves 6

Excellent with chicken or fish, this French vegetable stew is also wonderful served hot on a baked potato or even cold with crusty whole-grain bread. Ratatouille is best made a day ahead to allow some time for the flavors to blend.

1 teaspoon olive oil

2 medium onions, sliced

4 medium zucchini, cut into ½-inch slices

1 large eggplant, peeled (unless very young), cut into 1-inch cubes

2 large tomatoes, chopped

2 medium red, green, or yellow bell peppers, or any combination, chopped

1 tablespoon chopped fresh thyme or 1 teaspoon dried thyme, crumbled

1 tablespoon chopped fresh oregano or 1 teaspoon dried oregano, crumbled

1 tablespoon chopped fresh basil or 1 teaspoon dried basil, crumbled

2 medium garlic cloves, minced

⅛ teaspoon salt

Pepper to taste

In a large, heavy nonstick skillet, heat the oil over medium-high heat, swirling to coat the bottom. Cook the onions for 2 to 3 minutes, or until soft, stirring frequently.

Stir in the remaining ingredients. Reduce the heat and simmer, covered, for 30 to 45 minutes, or until the vegetables are cooked through, stirring occasionally to prevent sticking. Cook, uncovered, for 5 minutes to reduce the liquid.

Serve warm or cover and refrigerate to serve chilled.

PER SERVING

Calories 85	Cholesterol 0 mg	DIETARY EXCHANGES:
Total Fat 1.5 g	Sodium 67 mg	3 vegetable
Saturated Fat 0.5 g	Carbohydrates 17 g	½ fat
Trans Fat 0.0 g	Fiber 6 g	
Polyunsaturated Fat 0.5 g	Sugars 11 g	
Monounsaturated Fat 0.5 g	Protein 4 g	

Vegetable Pancakes

Serves 4

These Mexican-inspired pancakes are a different way to incorporate a variety of vegetables and make an interesting side dish for Pork with Corn-Cilantro Pesto (page 206) or Tilapia Tacos with Roasted-Tomato Salsa (page 128).

½ cup diced broccoli florets
½ cup diced cauliflower florets
½ cup diced mushrooms
½ cup diced onion (about 1 medium)
¼ cup diced red bell pepper
¼ cup egg substitute
¼ cup white whole-wheat flour
½ teaspoon baking powder
½ teaspoon chili powder
¼ teaspoon ground cumin
⅛ teaspoon salt
⅛ teaspoon pepper
1 teaspoon light tub margarine
1 teaspoon canola or corn oil

In a medium mixing bowl, combine the ingredients as follows: the broccoli, cauliflower, mushrooms, onion, bell pepper, egg substitute, flour, baking powder, chili powder, cumin, salt, and pepper.

In a large nonstick skillet, heat the margarine and oil over medium heat, swirling to coat the bottom. Using ¼ cup for each pancake, place 8 mounds of batter in the skillet (do this in batches if needed). Using a spatula, gently press down on the mounds to flatten them slightly. Cook the pancakes for 5 to 7 minutes on each side, or until browned.

COOK'S TIP: These pancakes can be made ahead of time and frozen. To reheat them, preheat the oven to 400°F. Put the frozen pancakes on a baking sheet. Bake them for 8 minutes (5 minutes if they're thawed).

PER SERVING

Calories 71	Cholesterol 0 mg	DIETARY EXCHANGES:
Total Fat 2.0 g	Sodium 180 mg	½ starch
Saturated Fat 0.0 g	Carbohydrates 11 g	1 vegetable
Trans Fat 0.0 g	Fiber 2 g	½ fat
Polyunsaturated Fat 0.5 g	Sugars 2 g	
Monounsaturated Fat 1.0 g	Protein 4 g	

Breads and Breakfast Dishes

ZUCCHINI BREAD 278

SPECKLED SPOON BREAD 280

CARDAMOM-LEMON MUFFINS 281

OATMEAL-FRUIT MUFFINS 282

PINEAPPLE-CARROT MUFFINS 284

PECAN-TOPPED CINNAMON OATMEAL 286

BLUEBERRY-YOGURT PANCAKES 287

PUFFED PANCAKE WITH APPLE-CRANBERRY SAUCE 288

BREAKFAST CROSTINI 290

BREAKFAST TORTILLA WRAP 291

FRENCH TOAST WITH PEACH AND PRALINE TOPPING 292

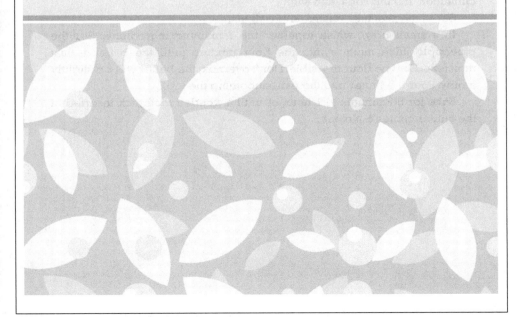

Zucchini Bread

Serves 16

The secret to this moist, flavorful, and healthy version of zucchini bread is pineapple juice, which replaces a lot of oil or butter that can add calories and too much saturated fat.

Cooking spray
1½ cups all-purpose flour
½ cup firmly packed light brown sugar
1½ teaspoons baking powder
½ teaspoon ground cinnamon
¼ teaspoon baking soda
⅛ teaspoon salt
1 cup shredded zucchini
¼ cup raisins
¼ cup finely chopped walnuts, dry-roasted
½ cup 100% pineapple juice
¼ cup egg substitute
1 tablespoon canola or corn oil
1 tablespoon light corn syrup
½ teaspoon vanilla extract

Preheat the oven to 350°F. Lightly spray a 9 x 5 x 3-inch loaf pan with cooking spray.

In a large bowl, stir together the flour, brown sugar, baking powder, cinnamon, baking soda, and salt.

Stir in the zucchini, raisins, and walnuts.

In a small bowl, whisk together the remaining ingredients. Stir the pineapple juice mixture into the flour mixture until the batter is just moistened but no flour is visible. Don't overmix; the batter will be slightly lumpy. Pour the batter into the pan, smoothing the top.

Bake for 50 minutes to 1 hour, or until a wooden toothpick inserted in the center comes out clean.

Transfer the pan to a cooling rack and let stand for 10 minutes. Using a spatula, loosen the bread from the side of the pan. Turn out onto the cooling rack. Let cool completely before slicing.

COOK'S TIP: Wrap leftovers in plastic wrap and refrigerate them for up to seven days.

PER SERVING

Calories 108	Cholesterol 0 mg	DIETARY EXCHANGES:
Total Fat 2.0 g	Sodium 87 mg	1½ starch
Saturated Fat 0.0 g	Carbohydrates 20 g	½ fat
Trans Fat 0.0 g	Fiber 1 g	
Polyunsaturated Fat 1.0 g	Sugars 10 g	
Monounsaturated Fat 0.5 g	Protein 2 g	

Speckled Spoon Bread

Serves 6

This soufflélike bread requires a spoon for serving and is dotted with corn, green onions, and pimiento.

Cooking spray
1 cup water
½ cup cornmeal
½ cup canned no-salt-added or frozen whole-kernel corn, thawed
¼ cup finely chopped green onions (green part only)
2 tablespoons chopped pimiento, patted dry
1 tablespoon light tub margarine
2 medium garlic cloves, minced
½ teaspoon salt-free all-purpose seasoning blend
⅛ teaspoon pepper
¾ cup fat-free milk
¼ cup egg substitute
1 teaspoon baking powder
3 large egg whites

Preheat the oven to 325°F. Lightly spray a 1½-quart glass casserole dish with cooking spray. Set aside.

In a medium saucepan, stir together the water and cornmeal. Bring to a boil over high heat. Reduce the heat to medium low. Cook for about 1 minute, or until very thick, stirring constantly. Remove from the heat. Stir in the corn, green onions, pimiento, margarine, garlic, seasoning blend, and pepper. Stir in the milk. In a small bowl, stir together the egg substitute and baking powder. Stir into the cornmeal mixture.

In a large stainless steel or glass mixing bowl, using an electric mixer on high speed, beat the egg whites until stiff peaks form (the peaks don't fall when the beaters are lifted). Fold into the cornmeal mixture, just until no whites show. Gently spoon into the baking dish. Bake for 50 minutes to 1 hour, or until a knife inserted near the center comes out clean.

PER SERVING

Calories 89	Cholesterol 1 mg	DIETARY EXCHANGES:
Total Fat 1.0 g	Sodium 147 mg	1 starch
Saturated Fat 0.0 g	Carbohydrates 16 g	½ lean meat
Trans Fat 0.0 g	Fiber 1 g	
Polyunsaturated Fat 0.5 g	Sugars 3 g	
Monounsaturated Fat 0.5 g	Protein 5 g	

Cardamom-Lemon Muffins

Serves 24

Cardamom adds a distinctive flavor to and enhances the sweetness of these muffins. Two kinds of whole grains bump up the fiber and applesauce keeps the muffins moist.

Cooking spray
2½ cups oat bran
2 cups white whole-wheat flour
2 teaspoons baking powder
1½ teaspoons baking soda
1 teaspoon ground cardamom
2 cups unsweetened applesauce
4 large egg whites
½ cup 100% pineapple juice
½ cup honey
2 tablespoons canola or corn oil
¼ teaspoon almond extract
2 to 3 teaspoons grated lemon zest

Preheat the oven to 400°F.

Lightly spray two standard 12-cup muffin pans with cooking spray.

In a large bowl, stir together the oat bran, flour, baking powder, baking soda, and cardamom.

In a separate large bowl, stir together the remaining ingredients. Stir the oat bran mixture into the applesauce mixture until the batter is just moistened but no flour is visible. Don't overmix; the batter will be lumpy. Spoon the batter into the muffin cups.

Put the pans in the oven. Reduce the temperature to 375°F. Bake for 18 to 20 minutes, or until golden brown.

Transfer the pans to a cooling rack. Let stand for 5 minutes. Serve the muffins warm or at room temperature.

PER SERVING

Calories 104	Cholesterol 0 mg	DIETARY EXCHANGES:
Total Fat 2.0 g	Sodium 122 mg	1½ starch
Saturated Fat 0.0 g	Carbohydrates 21 g	
Trans Fat 0.0 g	Fiber 3 g	
Polyunsaturated Fat 0.5 g	Sugars 9 g	
Monounsaturated Fat 1.0 g	Protein 4 g	

Oatmeal-Fruit Muffins

Serves 12

These wholesome muffins are packed with the goodness of whole grains. Dried fruit provides natural sweetness, so these have only a fraction of the added sugar found in most store-bought baked goods. Pair one with a glass of fat-free milk for a quick breakfast or healthy after-school snack.

Cooking spray
1 cup white whole-wheat flour
¾ cup uncooked oatmeal
⅓ cup toasted wheat germ
2 teaspoons baking powder
1 teaspoon ground cinnamon
½ teaspoon baking soda
⅛ teaspoon salt
¾ cup fat-free milk
½ cup firmly packed light brown sugar
¼ cup egg substitute
¼ cup unsweetened applesauce
½ teaspoon vanilla extract
½ cup chopped dried figs or dried apricots

Preheat the oven to 400°F. Lightly spray a standard 12-cup muffin pan with cooking spray.

In a medium bowl, stir together the flour, oatmeal, wheat germ, baking powder, cinnamon, baking soda, and salt.

In a separate medium bowl, stir together the remaining ingredients except the figs. Stir the milk mixture into the flour mixture until the batter is just moistened but no flour is visible. Don't overmix; the batter will be lumpy. Fold in the figs. Spoon the batter into the muffin cups.

Bake for 10 to 12 minutes, or until a wooden toothpick inserted in the center of a muffin comes out clean.

Transfer the pan to a cooling rack. Let stand for 5 minutes. Serve the muffins warm or at room temperature.

COOK'S TIP ON WHITE WHOLE-WHEAT FLOUR: White whole-wheat flour is made from hard white spring wheat, rather than the usual red wheat. It has a lower gluten content and lighter color, and it tastes more like refined white flour. Look for it in the baking or natural-foods aisle of your supermarket.

COOK'S TIP ON DRIED FRUIT: When buying dried fruit, be sure to choose products with no added sugar whenever possible.

PER SERVING

Calories 125	Cholesterol 0 mg	DIETARY EXCHANGES:
Total Fat 1.0 g	Sodium 164 mg	1½ starch
Saturated Fat 0.0 g	Carbohydrates 25 g	
Trans Fat 0.0 g	Fiber 3 g	
Polyunsaturated Fat 0.5 g	Sugars 14 g	
Monounsaturated Fat 0.0 g	Protein 4 g	

Pineapple-Carrot Muffins

Serves 12

These flavorful muffins are a great way to fit fruit and fiber into a portable breakfast treat. Fat-free yogurt adds moisture to baked goods without adding extra saturated fat.

Cooking spray
1 cup whole-wheat flour
1 cup unprocessed wheat bran
½ cup sugar
1 teaspoon baking soda
¾ teaspoon ground cinnamon
½ teaspoon baking powder
¼ teaspoon salt
6 ounces fat-free plain yogurt
2 tablespoons canola or corn oil
1 large egg white
1 teaspoon vanilla extract
1 8-ounce can crushed pineapple packed in its own juice, undrained
1 medium carrot, shredded

Preheat the oven to 400°F. Lightly spray a standard 12-cup muffin pan with cooking spray. Set aside.

In a large bowl, stir together the flour, wheat bran, sugar, baking soda, cinnamon, baking powder, and salt.

In a medium bowl, whisk together the yogurt, oil, egg white, and vanilla until well blended. Stir in the pineapple with liquid and the carrot. Stir the yogurt mixture into the flour mixture until the batter is just moistened but no flour is visible. Don't overmix; the batter will be lumpy. Spoon the batter into the muffin cups.

Bake for 18 to 20 minutes, or until a wooden toothpick inserted in the center of a muffin comes out clean.

Transfer the pan to a cooling rack. Let stand for at least 5 minutes. Serve the muffins warm or at room temperature.

COOK'S TIP ON UNPROCESSED WHEAT BRAN: Unprocessed wheat bran is the bran removed from wheat kernels. A very good source of fiber, it makes a healthy, flavorful addition to many foods, including meat loaf, burgers, and baked goods such as muffins, breads, and cookies. Health food stores and many supermarkets carry unprocessed wheat bran.

PER SERVING

Calories 121	Cholesterol 0 mg	DIETARY EXCHANGES:
Total Fat 3.0 g	Sodium 192 mg	1½ starch
Saturated Fat 0.0 g	Carbohydrates 22 g	
Trans Fat 0.0 g	Fiber 4 g	
Polyunsaturated Fat 1.0 g	Sugars 12 g	
Monounsaturated Fat 1.5 g	Protein 4 g	

Pecan-Topped Cinnamon Oatmeal

Serves 4

Start the day off right with this wholesome breakfast studded with cranberries and sprinkled with pecans and a blend of cinnamon and sugar, for just a hint of sweetness. Grated orange zest adds just a bit of fresh citrus flavor.

- 1 tablespoon plus 1 teaspoon sugar
- ¾ teaspoon ground cinnamon
- 2¾ cups fat-free milk
- 1½ cups uncooked oatmeal
- ⅓ cup sweetened dried cranberries
- ⅛ teaspoon salt
- 1 teaspoon grated orange zest
- 1 teaspoon light tub margarine
- ½ teaspoon vanilla extract or vanilla, butter, and nut flavoring
- 1 ounce finely chopped pecans, dry-roasted

In a small bowl, stir together the sugar and cinnamon. Set aside 2 teaspoons of the mixture for the topping.

In a large saucepan, bring the milk to a boil over medium-high heat. Stir in the oatmeal, cranberries, salt, and the sugar mixture from the small bowl. Reduce the heat and simmer for 5 minutes, stirring occasionally.

Stir in the orange zest, margarine, and vanilla. Let stand for 3 minutes so the flavors blend.

Transfer the oatmeal to bowls. Sprinkle with the pecans and the reserved 2 teaspoons sugar mixture.

PER SERVING

Calories 279	Cholesterol 3 mg	DIETARY EXCHANGES:
Total Fat 7.5 g	Sodium 152 mg	1½ starch
Saturated Fat 1.0 g	Carbohydrates 43 g	1 fat-free milk
Trans Fat 0.0 g	Fiber 4 g	½ fruit
Polyunsaturated Fat 2.5 g	Sugars 20 g	1 fat
Monounsaturated Fat 3.5 g	Protein 11 g	

Blueberry-Yogurt Pancakes

You get a whole serving of fruit in your first meal of the day with these pancakes. Drizzle them with pure maple syrup or scatter additional blueberries on top.

> 1½ cups white whole-wheat flour
> 1½ tablespoons sugar
> 1½ teaspoons baking powder
> ½ teaspoon ground nutmeg
> ¾ cup fat-free plain yogurt
> 1 large egg
> 2 tablespoons canola or corn oil and 1 teaspoon canola or corn oil, divided use
> 1 cup fat-free milk
> 2 cups blueberries (fresh preferred)

Preheat the oven to 200°F.

In a medium bowl, stir together the flour, sugar, baking powder, and nutmeg.

In a small bowl, whisk together the yogurt, egg, and 2 tablespoons oil. Slowly whisk in the milk.

Pour the yogurt mixture into the flour mixture. Stir just until blended but no flour is visible. Gently stir in the blueberries.

Heat a large nonstick griddle or skillet over medium heat until drops of water sprinkled on the griddle sizzle. Pour the remaining 1 teaspoon oil onto the griddle. Using a heatproof pastry brush, spread the oil over the surface.

Using a ⅓-cup measure, pour the batter for 6 pancakes onto the griddle. Cook the pancakes for 3 minutes, or until the bubbles on the tops have popped and the bottoms are golden brown. Turn over the pancakes. Cook for 1 minute, or until the bottoms are golden brown. Transfer the pancakes to a baking sheet, cover with aluminum foil, and put in the oven to keep warm while you cook the remaining batter.

PER SERVING

Calories 352	Cholesterol 49 mg	DIETARY EXCHANGES:
Total Fat 11.0 g	Sodium 231 mg	2½ starch
Saturated Fat 1.5 g	Carbohydrates 55 g	1 fruit
Trans Fat 0.0 g	Fiber 7 g	½ fat-free milk
Polyunsaturated Fat 3.0 g	Sugars 19 g	1½ fat
Monounsaturated Fat 6.0 g	Protein 13 g	

Puffed Pancake with Apple-Cranberry Sauce

Serves 6

Like French soufflés, German puffed pancakes should be served as soon as they're removed from the oven because they won't stay puffy for long. This dish would make an impressive addition to your next brunch, or serve it for a special weekend breakfast.

Cooking spray
2 teaspoons light tub margarine
¾ cup egg substitute
½ cup all-purpose flour
½ cup fat-free milk
⅛ teaspoon salt
2 large cooking apples, such as Rome Beauty, Golden Delicious, or Granny Smith, peeled, cored, and thinly sliced
¾ cup 100% apple juice and 2 tablespoons 100% apple juice, divided use
½ cup fresh or frozen unsweetened cranberries or blackberries, thawed if frozen
¼ cup sugar
¼ teaspoon ground cinnamon
1 tablespoon cornstarch

Preheat the oven to 400°F.

Lightly spray a medium ovenproof skillet with cooking spray. Add the margarine. Put the skillet in the oven for 3 minutes, or until the margarine is melted.

In a medium mixing bowl, using an electric mixer on medium speed or a wire whisk, beat together the egg substitute, flour, milk, and salt until smooth. Immediately pour the mixture into the hot skillet. Bake for about 25 minutes, or until puffy and brown.

Meanwhile, in a medium skillet, stir together the apples, ¾ cup apple juice, cranberries, sugar, and cinnamon. Bring to a boil over high heat. Reduce the heat and simmer, covered, for about 10 minutes, or until the fruit is tender, stirring occasionally.

Put the cornstarch in a small bowl. Add the remaining 2 tablespoons apple juice, whisking to dissolve. Stir into the apple mixture. Cook for about 2 minutes, or until thickened and bubbly, stirring frequently.

Just before serving, cut the pancake into wedges. Spoon the sauce over each serving.

COOK'S TIP: The apple-cranberry sauce can be made in advance. Reheat it in a small saucepan over low heat, stirring occasionally. Or put the sauce in a microwaveable cup or bowl and microwave, loosely covered, on 100 percent power (high) for 1 to 2 minutes, stirring twice during the cooking time.

PER SERVING

Calories 157	Cholesterol 0 mg	DIETARY EXCHANGES:
Total Fat 1.0 g	Sodium 132 mg	1½ starch
Saturated Fat 0.0 g	Carbohydrates 34 g	1 fruit
Trans Fat 0.0 g	Fiber 2 g	
Polyunsaturated Fat 0.0 g	Sugars 21 g	
Monounsaturated Fat 0.5 g	Protein 5 g	

Breakfast Crostini

Serves 4

In Italian, *crostini* means "little toasts," and they are usually served as an appetizer. These egg-and-vegetable toasts, however, are a nutritious way to energize your morning with a boost of protein.

   1 **teaspoon light tub margarine**
  ¼ **cup chopped button mushrooms**
  1 **tablespoon minced fresh parsley**
  1 **tablespoon minced green onions (green part only)**
  ⅛ **teaspoon pepper**
  ¾ **cup egg substitute**
  4 **slices light whole-wheat bread (lowest sodium available)**
  ¼ **cup chopped, seeded tomato**

In a medium nonstick skillet, melt the margarine over medium heat, swirling to coat the bottom. Cook the mushrooms for about 2 minutes, or until tender, stirring frequently. Sprinkle with the parsley, green onions, and pepper. Reduce the heat to low. Pour the egg substitute into the skillet. Cook for about 2 minutes, or until the egg substitute is cooked and set, stirring frequently. Remove from the heat.

Toast the bread. Spoon the egg substitute mixture onto the toast. Cut in half diagonally. Sprinkle with the tomato.

PER SERVING

Calories 70	Cholesterol 0 mg	DIETARY EXCHANGES:
Total Fat 0.5 g	Sodium 218 mg	½ starch
Saturated Fat 0.0 g	Carbohydrates 11 g	1 lean meat
Trans Fat 0.0 g	Fiber 4 g	
Polyunsaturated Fat 0.0 g	Sugars 3 g	
Monounsaturated Fat 0.0 g	Protein 7 g	

Breakfast Tortilla Wrap

Serves 4

These wraps are a hearty breakfast in a grab-and-go package. Scrambled egg whites are layered with a mixture of potatoes and Canadian bacon, topped with cheese, and rolled in a corn tortilla.

- **4 large egg whites, lightly beaten**
- **⅛ teaspoon pepper and ⅛ teaspoon pepper, divided use**
- **1 cup frozen fat-free shredded potatoes**
- **½ medium red bell pepper, diced**
- **1 ounce Canadian bacon, chopped**
- **1 teaspoon canola or corn oil**
- **4 6-inch corn tortillas**
- **¼ cup shredded low-fat Cheddar cheese**

In a small nonstick skillet, cook the egg whites and ⅛ teaspoon pepper over medium-low heat for 3 to 4 minutes, or until cooked through, stirring occasionally. Set aside.

Meanwhile, in a medium bowl, stir together the potatoes, bell pepper, Canadian bacon, and the remaining ⅛ teaspoon pepper.

In a medium nonstick skillet, heat the oil over medium-high heat, swirling to coat the bottom. Spread the potato mixture evenly in the skillet. Cook for 6 to 7 minutes on one side, or until the potatoes are a light golden brown. Using a spatula, turn over the potato mixture. Cook for 5 to 6 minutes, or until light golden brown.

Meanwhile, warm the tortillas using the package directions. Transfer the tortillas to a work surface.

Layer as follows in the center of the tortillas: the egg whites, the potato mixture, and the Cheddar. Roll up jelly-roll style, starting at the bottom. Secure with a wooden toothpick, if desired.

Serve immediately or refrigerate in an airtight container or individually wrapped in plastic wrap. To reheat, place 1 or 2 wraps on a microwaveable plate. Microwave on 100 percent power (high) for 1 to 1½ minutes, or until heated through.

PER SERVING

Calories 124	Cholesterol 5 mg	DIETARY EXCHANGES:
Total Fat 2.5 g	Sodium 228 mg	1 starch
Saturated Fat 0.5 g	Carbohydrates 17 g	1 lean meat
Trans Fat 0.0 g	Fiber 2 g	
Polyunsaturated Fat 0.5 g	Sugars 1 g	
Monounsaturated Fat 1.0 g	Protein 9 g	

French Toast with Peach and Praline Topping

Serves 8

This version of French toast is sweet and crunchy, thanks to southern accents from peaches and pecans.

- 1 **cup fat-free milk**
- 4 **large egg whites**
- ½ **teaspoon ground cinnamon and ¼ teaspoon ground cinnamon, divided use**
- 8 **slices reduced-calorie whole-grain bread (lowest sodium available)**
- 1 **teaspoon canola or corn oil and 1 teaspoon canola or corn oil, divided use**
- 1 **15-ounce can sliced peaches in juice, undrained**
- ⅓ **cup chopped pecans, dry-roasted**
- 2 **tablespoons light brown sugar**
- 1 **tablespoon fresh lemon juice**
- 1 **teaspoon vanilla extract**
- ¼ **teaspoon ground nutmeg**

Preheat the oven to 200°F. In a medium shallow bowl, whisk together the milk, egg whites, and ½ teaspoon cinnamon. Working quickly with half the bread, lightly dip in the milk mixture, turning to coat. Transfer to a large plate. Repeat with the remaining bread and milk mixture.

Using a nonstick griddle over medium heat, heat 1 teaspoon oil, swirling to coat the griddle. Cook half the bread for 2 to 3 minutes on each side, or until golden brown. Transfer to a baking sheet and put in the oven to keep warm while you cook the remaining bread, using the remaining 1 teaspoon oil.

In a medium saucepan, stir together the peaches with juice, pecans, brown sugar, lemon juice, vanilla, nutmeg, and the remaining ¼ teaspoon cinnamon. Bring to a simmer over medium-high heat. Reduce the heat and simmer for 3 to 4 minutes so the flavors blend, stirring occasionally. Transfer the French toast to plates. Spoon the topping over the French toast.

PER SERVING

Calories 151	Cholesterol 1 mg	DIETARY EXCHANGES:
Total Fat 5.0 g	Sodium 165 mg	1 starch
Saturated Fat 0.5 g	Carbohydrates 23 g	½ fruit
Trans Fat 0.0 g	Fiber 5 g	½ lean meat
Polyunsaturated Fat 1.5 g	Sugars 12 g	½ fat
Monounsaturated Fat 2.5 g	Protein 5 g	

Desserts

LEMON POPPY SEED CAKE 294

PUMPKIN-CARROT CAKE 296

CHOCOLATE MINI-CHEESECAKES 297

APPLE-RHUBARB CRISP 298

CHERRY-PEAR TURNOVERS 300

FRESH PEACH AND GINGER CRISP 302

GINGERSNAP AND GRAHAM CRACKER CRUST 303

MAPLE-BLUEBERRY BARS 304

MOCK BAKLAVA 306

NUTTY MERINGUE KISSES 307

COCONUT CORNFLAKE COOKIES 308

CHOCOLATE SOUFFLÉS WITH VANILLA SAUCE 309

MANGO BRÛLÉE WITH PINE NUTS 310

HONEY-BAKED PECAN PEACHES 311

CREPES SUZETTE WITH RASPBERRIES 312

APPLE-RAISIN SAUCE 314

BANANAS FOSTER PLUS 315

STRAWBERRIES ROMANOFF 316

VERY BERRY SORBET 317

STRAWBERRY MARGARITA ICE 318

Lemon Poppy Seed Cake

Serves 10

Perfect with an afternoon cup of tea, this moist cake—thanks to plenty of applesauce—has a bold lemon flavor accented with the delicate crunch of poppy seeds.

> **Cooking spray**
> 2 **cups all-purpose flour**
> ⅓ **cup sugar**
> 1 **tablespoon poppy seeds**
> 1½ **teaspoons baking powder**
> ¼ **teaspoon baking soda**
> ⅛ **teaspoon salt**
> ¾ **cup unsweetened applesauce**
> 1 **teaspoon grated lemon zest**
> ¼ **cup fresh lemon juice**
> 3 **tablespoons canola or corn oil**
> 1 **tablespoon light corn syrup**
> 1 **teaspoon lemon extract**
> 4 **large egg whites**

Preheat the oven to 350°F. Lightly spray a 9-inch round cake pan with cooking spray.

In a medium bowl, stir together the flour, sugar, poppy seeds, baking powder, baking soda, and salt.

In a separate medium bowl, whisk together the remaining ingredients except the egg whites. Stir into the flour mixture until the batter is just moistened and no flour is visible.

In a large stainless steel or glass mixing bowl, using an electric mixer on high speed, beat the egg whites until stiff peaks form (the peaks don't fall when the beaters are lifted).

Using a rubber scraper, gently fold the batter into the beaten egg whites. Pour into the cake pan, lightly smoothing the top with the scraper.

Bake for 30 minutes, or until a wooden toothpick inserted in the center comes out clean. Let cool in the pan for 10 minutes. Loosen the sides of the cake with a thin metal spatula. Invert the cake onto a cooling rack. Serve warm, at room temperature, or chilled.

COOK'S TIP ON POPPY SEEDS AND SESAME SEEDS: You can intensify the flavor of both poppy and sesame seeds by dry-roasting them. Store these tasty and useful seeds in the refrigerator. Otherwise, the oil in the seeds can turn rancid and ruin them.

PER SERVING

Calories 183
Total Fat 5.0 g
  Saturated Fat 0.5 g
  Trans Fat 0.0 g
  Polyunsaturated Fat 1.5 g
  Monounsaturated Fat 2.5 g

Cholesterol 0 mg
Sodium 145 mg
Carbohydrates 31 g
  Fiber 1 g
  Sugars 11 g
Protein 4 g

DIETARY EXCHANGES:
2 other carbohydrate
1 fat

Pumpkin-Carrot Cake

Serves 8

When the days grow cooler and the kids have headed back to school, it's pumpkin time. Whip up this spicy, from-scratch cake as a warm, welcome-home snack or tuck slices into their lunch boxes.

Cooking spray
1 cup finely grated carrots
½ cup canned solid-pack pumpkin (not pie filling)
½ cup egg substitute
1 tablespoon canola or corn oil
1 teaspoon vanilla extract
1 cup white whole-wheat flour
⅓ cup sugar
¼ cup chopped walnuts
1 teaspoon ground cinnamon
1 teaspoon ground ginger
1 teaspoon pumpkin pie spice
½ teaspoon baking soda

Preheat the oven to 350°F. Lightly spray an 8-inch square metal baking pan with cooking spray.

In a medium bowl, whisk together the carrots, pumpkin, egg substitute, oil, and vanilla.

In a small bowl, stir together the remaining ingredients. Stir into the carrot mixture just until combined but no flour is visible. Spoon into the baking pan. Bake for 25 to 30 minutes, or until a wooden toothpick inserted in the center comes out clean. Transfer to a cooling rack and let cool for at least 15 minutes.

....

cook's tip: For this recipe, be sure to use finely grated carrots and not the shredded carrots sold in the grocery store, which are thicker and drier than carrots you grate yourself.

....

PER SERVING

Calories 145	Cholesterol 0 mg	DIETARY EXCHANGES:
Total Fat 4.5 g	Sodium 120 mg	1½ other carbohydrate
Saturated Fat 0.5 g	Carbohydrates 21 g	1 fat
Trans Fat 0.0 g	Fiber 3 g	
Polyunsaturated Fat 2.5 g	Sugars 11 g	
Monounsaturated Fat 1.5 g	Protein 5 g	

Chocolate Mini-Cheesecakes

Serves 12

Each of these mini-cheesecakes is a near perfect 100-calorie dessert, so no need to feel guilty for indulging in this sumptuous treat. Good things really do come in small packages!

¼ cup plus 2 tablespoons chocolate graham cracker crumbs

4 ounces low-fat cream cheese, softened

4 ounces fat-free cream cheese, softened

½ cup sugar

½ cup fat-free sour cream

½ cup egg substitute

2 tablespoons unsweetened cocoa powder

1 teaspoon vanilla extract

Preheat the oven to 325°F.

Line a standard 12-cup muffin pan with foil or paper bake cups. Sprinkle 1½ teaspoons crumbs into each.

In a large mixing bowl, using an electric mixer on medium-high speed, beat the cream cheeses, sugar, and sour cream until light and fluffy, about 3 minutes.

Add the egg substitute, cocoa powder, and vanilla. Beat on medium speed until blended. Fill the bake cups with the mixture (an ice cream scoop works well for this).

Bake for 18 to 20 minutes, or until the centers are set (the cheesecakes don't jiggle when gently shaken). Transfer the pan to a cooling rack and let cool for 15 to 20 minutes. Cover the pan and refrigerate for at least 30 minutes, or until completely cooled, before serving.

PER SERVING

Calories 95	Cholesterol 9 mg	DIETARY EXCHANGES:
Total Fat 2.0 g	Sodium 161 mg	1 other carbohydrate
Saturated Fat 1.0 g	Carbohydrates 15 g	
Trans Fat 0.0 g	Fiber 0 g	
Polyunsaturated Fat 0.0 g	Sugars 11 g	
Monounsaturated Fat 0.5 g	Protein 4 g	

Apple-Rhubarb Crisp

Serves 8

The apples help to sweeten up rhubarb's extreme tartness in this classic dessert that's perfect for crisp fall and winter evenings.

Cooking spray

FILLING

2 cups sliced fresh or frozen unsweetened rhubarb, thawed and drained if frozen

2 cups cored, peeled, and sliced cooking apples, such as Rome Beauty, Winesap, or Granny Smith

½ cup sugar

1 tablespoon cornstarch

TOPPING

⅔ cup uncooked regular or quick-cooking oatmeal

½ cup white whole-wheat flour

¼ cup firmly packed light brown sugar

3½ tablespoons light tub margarine

Lightly spray an 8-inch square glass baking dish or 1-quart glass casserole dish with cooking spray. Put the filling ingredients in the dish and stir together. Let stand for 1 hour.

Preheat the oven to 375°F.

In a medium bowl, stir together the oatmeal, flour, and brown sugar.

Using a pastry blender, cut the margarine into the topping mixture until it resembles coarse crumbs. Sprinkle over the filling.

Bake for 30 to 40 minutes, or until the topping is light brown. Transfer the dish to a cooling rack and let cool for about 20 minutes before serving.

....

COOK'S TIP ON CORING APPLES: If you don't have an apple corer, halve the fruit and use either a melon baller or a sturdy, rounded metal ½-teaspoon measuring spoon to scoop out the core and seeds.

....

COOK'S TIP ON RHUBARB: When buying fresh rhubarb, look for sturdy, brightly colored stalks. The leaves (which are inedible because they contain oxalic acid, which is toxic if ingested) should look fresh and be free of blemishes. To store rhubarb, wrap it tightly in plastic wrap or put it in a plastic bag, then refrigerate it for up to three days. Remove and discard the leaves just before using the stalks. Although most frequently eaten in combination with fruits, botanically speaking, rhubarb is considered a vegetable.

PER SERVING

Calories 166	Cholesterol 0 mg	DIETARY EXCHANGES:
Total Fat 2.5 g	Sodium 43 mg	2½ other carbohydrate
Saturated Fat 0.0 g	Carbohydrates 34 g	½ fat
Trans Fat 0.0 g	Fiber 2 g	
Polyunsaturated Fat 0.5 g	Sugars 23 g	
Monounsaturated Fat 1.5 g	Protein 2 g	

Cherry-Pear Turnovers

Serves 8

Phyllo dough, a healthier alternative to butter-laden crusts, envelops a mixed-fruit filling in these flaky turnovers. Whether you eat them with your hands or use a fork, they are a tasty way to end a meal.

Cooking spray

FILLING

1 14.5-ounce can tart cherries packed in water, undrained
1 medium Anjou or Bartlett pear, halved and chopped
⅓ cup sweetened dried cranberries or raisins
¼ cup frozen 100% apple juice concentrate, thawed
2½ tablespoons cornstarch
2 tablespoons plus 1 teaspoon sugar
1¼ teaspoons almond extract

PASTRY

8 sheets frozen phyllo dough (each 9 x 14 inches), thawed
2 teaspoons sugar
¾ teaspoon ground cinnamon

Preheat the oven to 400°F. Lightly spray a baking sheet with cooking spray. Set aside.

In a large saucepan, stir together the filling ingredients except the almond extract. Bring to a boil over medium-high heat. Boil for 1 minute, stirring once or twice. Remove from the heat. Stir in the almond extract. Let stand for 10 minutes to cool slightly.

Keeping the unused phyllo covered with a damp cloth or damp paper towels to prevent drying, lay one sheet of phyllo with the shorter side toward you on a flat work surface. Working quickly, lightly spray both sides of the phyllo sheet with cooking spray. Fold the sheet in half (to form a 9 x 7-inch sheet). Spoon ⅓ cup cherry mixture onto the sheet near the bottom. Roll up the sheet, folding in the sides as you go, to resemble an egg roll. Place with the seam side down on the baking sheet. Repeat with the remaining phyllo and filling.

In a small bowl, stir together the cinnamon and the remaining 2 teaspoons sugar. Sprinkle over the turnovers.

Bake for 16 minutes, or until golden. Transfer the baking sheet to a cooling rack and let cool for at least 1 hour so the flavors blend. Serve the same day for peak flavor and texture.

COOK'S TIP ON PEARS: To see if a pear is ripe, press gently on the neck near the stem. There should be a slight give. If your pear is too firm, let it stand at room temperature until it's ripe. To hasten ripening, place the pear in a paper bag with an apple, then let it stand at room temperature.

PER SERVING

Calories 129	Cholesterol 0 mg	DIETARY EXCHANGES:
Total Fat 0.5 g	Sodium 52 mg	1½ fruit
Saturated Fat 0.0 g	Carbohydrates 31 g	½ starch
Trans Fat 0.0 g	Fiber 2 g	
Polyunsaturated Fat 0.0 g	Sugars 18 g	
Monounsaturated Fat 0.0 g	Protein 1 g	

Fresh Peach and Ginger Crisp

Serves 9

Crystallized ginger boosts the flavor in this sweet, crunchy fruit crisp, elevating this version from the traditional one.

Cooking spray

FILLING

3 pounds peaches, peeled and sliced
2 tablespoons sugar
1½ tablespoons cornstarch
1½ tablespoons minced crystallized ginger

TOPPING

1 cup uncooked quick-cooking oatmeal
⅓ cup finely chopped pecans
¼ cup whole-wheat flour
¼ cup firmly packed light brown sugar
1 teaspoon ground cinnamon
1 tablespoon minced crystallized ginger
3 tablespoons fat-free milk
1 tablespoon canola or corn oil

Preheat the oven to 350°F. Lightly spray an 8-inch square baking pan with cooking spray.

In a medium bowl, stir together the filling ingredients. Spoon into the pan.

In a separate medium bowl, using a fork, stir together the oatmeal, pecans, flour, brown sugar, cinnamon, and the remaining 1 tablespoon ginger. Gradually add the milk and oil, stirring until the mixture is moistened. Sprinkle over the filling.

Bake for 30 minutes, or until the peaches are tender and the topping is golden brown. Transfer the pan to a cooling rack. Let cool for about 30 minutes. Serve warm. Cover and refrigerate any leftovers for up to two days.

PER SERVING

Calories 200	Cholesterol 0 mg	DIETARY EXCHANGES:
Total Fat 5.5 g	Sodium 5 mg	½ starch
Saturated Fat 0.5 g	Carbohydrates 37 g	1 fruit
Trans Fat 0.0 g	Fiber 4 g	1 other carbohydrate
Polyunsaturated Fat 1.5 g	Sugars 23 g	1 fat
Monounsaturated Fat 3.0 g	Protein 4 g	

Gingersnap and Graham Cracker Crust

Serves 8

You don't have to weigh your pie down with all that dough full of saturated and trans fats. Instead, go lighter with this crumb crust; it's a perfect balance of lightly spicy and lightly sweet.

- ¾ **cup low-fat graham cracker crumbs**
- ¾ **cup low-fat gingersnap crumbs**
- 2 **tablespoons light corn syrup**
- 2 **tablespoons 100% apple juice**

In a medium bowl, stir together all the ingredients. Using your fingers, press the mixture onto the bottom and up the side of a 9-inch pie pan.

The crust is ready to fill and bake. If you need a prebaked crust, bake it at 350°F for 10 minutes, then let cool before filling.

PER SERVING

Calories 89	Cholesterol 0 mg	DIETARY EXCHANGES:
Total Fat 1.5 g	Sodium 78 mg	1 other carbohydrate
Saturated Fat 0.5 g	Carbohydrates 18 g	
Trans Fat 0.0 g	Fiber 0 g	
Polyunsaturated Fat 0.0 g	Sugars 10 g	
Monounsaturated Fat 0.5 g	Protein 1 g	

Maple-Blueberry Bars

Serves 12

Love blueberry pie? These rich, fruit-filled bars will satisfy your craving without all that work, while helping you avoid saturated and trans fats. They're also low in added sugar.

- 2 cups fresh or frozen unsweetened blueberries, thawed if frozen
- 1 tablespoon pure maple syrup and 1 tablespoon pure maple syrup, divided use
- 1 tablespoon cornstarch
- 1 teaspoon grated lemon zest
- 1 tablespoon fresh lemon juice
- 1 teaspoon vanilla extract
- Cooking spray
- ¾ cup almond flour
- ¾ cup uncooked regular or quick-cooking oatmeal
- 3 tablespoons light brown sugar
- ⅓ cup low-fat buttermilk
- 2 tablespoons fat-free plain Greek yogurt
- 1 large egg white

In a small saucepan, stir together the blueberries, 1 tablespoon maple syrup, the cornstarch, lemon zest, lemon juice, and vanilla. Bring to a simmer over medium-high heat. Reduce the heat and simmer for 5 minutes, or until the blueberries are tender and the mixture is thickened, gently stirring occasionally if you want a chunky texture (no need to be gentle if you want the blueberries more mashed). Remove from the heat. Set aside.

Preheat the oven to 350°F. Lightly spray a 9-inch square metal baking pan with cooking spray.

In a medium bowl, stir together the almond flour, oatmeal, and brown sugar.

Stir in the remaining ingredients just until combined but no flour is visible. Don't overmix; the batter should be lumpy. Reserve ⅓ cup mixture for the topping.

To assemble, spread the remaining mixture in the baking pan. Spread the blueberry mixture on top. Using your hands, crumble the reserved topping mixture over the blueberry mixture.

Bake for 30 minutes, or until the topping is lightly browned. Transfer to a cooling rack and let cool for 15 minutes before cutting into bars.

COOK'S TIP ON ALMOND FLOUR: Almond flour, also called almond meal, is made from blanched almonds ground into a fine powder. Look for it in the natural-foods aisle of the grocery store.

PER SERVING

Calories 109	Cholesterol 0 mg	DIETARY EXCHANGES:
Total Fat 4.5 g	Sodium 14 mg	1 other carbohydrate
Saturated Fat 0.5 g	Carbohydrates 15 g	1 fat
Trans Fat 0.0 g	Fiber 2 g	
Polyunsaturated Fat 1.5 g	Sugars 9 g	
Monounsaturated Fat 2.0 g	Protein 3 g	

Mock Baklava

Serves 12

Traditional baklava is usually full of butter and, therefore, saturated fat. Thanks to butter-flavor cooking spray, here is a revamped and no-guilt version of this Greek sweet.

> ¾ cup raisins
> ⅔ cup finely chopped pecans or walnuts, dry-roasted
> Butter-flavor cooking spray
> 8 sheets frozen phyllo dough, thawed
> ½ cup honey
> 2 teaspoons ground cinnamon

Preheat the oven to 350°F.

In a small bowl, stir together the raisins and pecans.

Lightly spraying every other phyllo sheet with cooking spray, stack the sheets on a work surface. Working quickly, spread the raisin-nut mixture over the top sheet, leaving a 1-inch border on all sides.

Drizzle with the honey and sprinkle with the cinnamon.

Starting on a long side, roll lengthwise, jelly-roll style. Tucking the ends of the roll under, place with the seam side down on a nonstick baking sheet. Lightly spray the top with cooking spray. Cut shallow slashes through the pastry to the raisin-nut mixture at 1½-inch intervals so steam can escape during baking.

Bake for 20 to 30 minutes, or until light golden brown. Cut into 12 slices using the vent lines as guides.

....

COOK'S TIP: This dish freezes well. Prepare as directed but omit spraying the top and baking. (Do cut the steam vents.) Freeze overnight on a baking sheet, then wrap in freezer paper or aluminum foil for freezing. To bake, place the frozen baklava on a nonstick baking sheet, lightly spray with butter-flavor cooking spray, and bake at 350°F for 35 to 45 minutes, or until golden brown.

....

PER SERVING

Calories 164	Cholesterol 0 mg	DIETARY EXCHANGES:
Total Fat 5.0 g	Sodium 63 mg	2 other carbohydrate
Saturated Fat 0.5 g	Carbohydrates 31 g	1 fat
Trans Fat 0.0 g	Fiber 2 g	
Polyunsaturated Fat 1.5 g	Sugars 18 g	
Monounsaturated Fat 2.5 g	Protein 2 g	

Nutty Meringue Kisses

Serves 8

These meringues are crisp, airy, and filled with nutty goodness. They take some time, because they bake at a very low temperature for two hours and then stand in the oven for another two hours. You'll need to plan ahead, but you'll be very glad you did.

4 **large egg whites**
¼ **teaspoon cream of tartar**
¼ **cup pure maple syrup**
1 **teaspoon vanilla extract**
⅓ **cup finely chopped pecans or walnuts**

Preheat the oven to 200°F. Line two large baking sheets with cooking parchment.

In a large stainless steel or glass mixing bowl, using an electric mixer on high speed, beat the egg whites and cream of tartar until stiff peaks form (the peaks don't fall when the beaters are lifted).

Add the maple syrup and vanilla, a little at a time, beating well after each addition. Fold in the pecans.

Spoon the batter into a large resealable plastic bag. Using scissors, cut off a bottom corner of the bag. Squeeze the batter onto the parchment in small dollops.

Bake for 2 hours. Turn off the oven, leaving the baking sheets inside and the oven door closed. Let the cookies stand in the oven for 2 hours. Store in an airtight container for up to three days.

PER SERVING

Calories 68	Cholesterol 0 mg	DIETARY EXCHANGES:
Total Fat 3.5 g	Sodium 29 mg	½ other carbohydrate
Saturated Fat 0.5 g	Carbohydrates 8 g	½ fat
Trans Fat 0.0 g	Fiber 0 g	
Polyunsaturated Fat 1.0 g	Sugars 7 g	
Monounsaturated Fat 2.0 g	Protein 2 g	

Coconut Cornflake Cookies

Serves 30

Adults and children alike will be so hooked on these crunchy, fruity cornflake nuggets that you'll want to serve them for breakfast, too!

Cooking spray
1 **cup sugar**
⅔ **cup light tub margarine, at room temperature**
½ **cup egg substitute**
1 **teaspoon vanilla extract**
1 **teaspoon coconut extract**
3 **cups all-purpose flour**
1 **teaspoon baking powder**
½ **teaspoon baking soda**
1 **cup dried mixed fruit bits**
2 **cups coarsely crushed cornflake cereal**

Preheat the oven to 375°F. Lightly spray two baking sheets with cooking spray.

In a large bowl, stir together the sugar, margarine, egg substitute, and vanilla and coconut extracts until smooth.

In a small bowl, combine the flour, baking powder, and baking soda. Using a spoon, gradually stir into the sugar mixture until the flour is incorporated (the dough will be slightly sticky).

Gently stir in the fruit bits to distribute throughout the dough.

Put the cornflakes in a shallow bowl or on a large platter. Drop a teaspoon of dough onto the cornflakes and roll to coat. Place the cookie on a baking sheet and flatten slightly with the bottom of a glass. Repeat with the remaining dough, leaving 2 inches between cookies.

Bake for 10 to 11 minutes, or until the cookies feel slightly soft when lightly pressed in the center. Transfer the cookies to cooling racks. Let cool completely, about 30 minutes.

PER SERVING

Calories 118	Cholesterol 0 mg	DIETARY EXCHANGES:
Total Fat 1.5 g	Sodium 110 mg	1½ other carbohydrate
Saturated Fat 0.0 g	Carbohydrates 23 g	½ fat
Trans Fat 0.0 g	Fiber 1 g	
Polyunsaturated Fat 0.5 g	Sugars 10 g	
Monounsaturated Fat 1.0 g	Protein 2 g	

Chocolate Soufflés with Vanilla Sauce

Serves 6

These light-as-air soufflés use cocoa powder instead of chocolate, and add a hint of bittersweet orange flavor. One spoonful and you'll forget you're not eating their beloved, high-fat counterpart.

Cooking spray
⅓ cup fresh orange juice
¼ cup sugar
4 large egg whites
¼ cup unsweetened cocoa powder (Dutch-process preferred)
2 tablespoons orange liqueur or fresh orange juice
¾ cup fat-free, sugar-free vanilla ice cream or frozen yogurt, softened

Preheat the oven to 300°F. Lightly spray six 5- or 6-ounce custard cups with cooking spray. Set aside.

In a small saucepan, whisk together the orange juice and sugar. Cook over medium-high heat for 3 to 4 minutes, or until the mixture is syrupy, whisking occasionally. Remove from the heat.

In a large stainless steel or glass mixing bowl, using an electric mixer on high speed, beat the egg whites until stiff peaks form (the peaks don't fall when the beaters are lifted). Pour the syrup over the egg whites. Beat for 2 minutes. Add the cocoa and liqueur. Beat just until well blended. Pour into the custard cups.

Bake for 12 minutes, or until the soufflés have puffed. Don't overbake or the soufflés will become tough.

Just before serving, spoon 2 tablespoons softened ice cream into the center of each soufflé. Serve immediately.

....

COOK'S TIP ON BEATING EGG WHITES: Even a drop of yolk will prevent egg whites from forming peaks when beaten, so separate eggs very carefully.

....

PER SERVING

Calories 102	Cholesterol 0 mg	DIETARY EXCHANGES:
Total Fat 0.5 g	Sodium 50 mg	1½ other carbohydrate
Saturated Fat 0.0 g	Carbohydrates 19 g	
Trans Fat 0.0 g	Fiber 1 g	
Polyunsaturated Fat 0.0 g	Sugars 13 g	
Monounsaturated Fat 0.0 g	Protein 4 g	

Mango Brûlée with Pine Nuts

Serves 4

This heart-healthy version of crème brûlée, which literally means "burned cream," starts with golden cubes of tart and tangy tropical fruit and then is topped with a layer of fat-free sour cream for its richness. The dessert is finished with crunchy nuts and brown sugar that is caramelized under the broiler.

2 cups cubed mango, papaya, or peaches
⅔ cup fat-free sour cream
2 tablespoons pine nuts
2 tablespoons dark brown sugar

Preheat the broiler.

Arrange the fruit in a single layer in a 9-inch pie pan.

Dollop with the sour cream. Spread the sour cream into an even layer.

Sprinkle the pine nuts and brown sugar over the sour cream.

Broil 4 to 6 inches from the heat for 1 to 2 minutes, or until the sugar melts and the pine nuts are toasted. Watch carefully so they don't burn. Serve immediately.

....

COOK'S TIP: If fresh fruit is out of season, you can use frozen unsweetened fruit that's been thawed, fruit in a jar, or fruit canned in 100 percent juice.

....

PER SERVING

Calories 135	Cholesterol 7 mg	DIETARY EXCHANGES:
Total Fat 2.0 g	Sodium 36 mg	1 fruit
Saturated Fat 0.5 g	Carbohydrates 26 g	1 other carbohydrate
Trans Fat 0.0 g	Fiber 2 g	½ fat
Polyunsaturated Fat 1.0 g	Sugars 21 g	
Monounsaturated Fat 1.0 g	Protein 4 g	

Honey-Baked Pecan Peaches

Serves 8

Fresh fruit takes on a whole new flavor when it's baked. Drizzle it with a warm mixture of cinnamon, honey, and nuts, and this dessert skyrockets from good to great.

Cooking spray
2 **tablespoons honey**
¼ **cup finely chopped pecans**
¼ **teaspoon ground cinnamon**
4 **large peaches or nectarines (about 6 ounces each), peeled if desired and halved**
2 **tablespoons light tub margarine**
¼ **teaspoon vanilla extract**

Preheat the oven to 350°F.

Lightly spray a 9-inch round cake or pie pan with cooking spray. Pour the honey into the pan and heat in the oven for 2 minutes, or until the honey is the consistency of pancake syrup. Remove the pan from the oven, swirling to coat the bottom.

Sprinkle the pecans over the honey.

Sprinkle the cinnamon over the cut sides of the peaches. Place with the cut side down on the pecans. Using a fork, pierce each peach half several times for faster cooking.

Bake for 20 minutes, or until the peaches are tender. Leaving the syrup in the pan, transfer the peaches with the cut side up to a platter.

Add the margarine and vanilla to the syrup, stirring until the margarine melts. Spoon over the peaches. Let stand for 10 minutes so the flavors blend. Serve warm or at room temperature.

PER SERVING

Calories 84	Cholesterol 0 mg	DIETARY EXCHANGES:
Total Fat 4.0 g	Sodium 23 mg	1 other carbohydrate
Saturated Fat 0.0 g	Carbohydrates 13 g	1 fat
Trans Fat 0.0 g	Fiber 2 g	
Polyunsaturated Fat 1.0 g	Sugars 12 g	
Monounsaturated Fat 2.0 g	Protein 1 g	

Crepes Suzette with Raspberries

Serves 8

The orange-raspberry sauce is an extraordinary topping for the thin French pancakes known as crepes, and this healthful version has less fat and sugar than the traditional ones.

CREPES

1¼ cups fat-free milk

¾ cup white whole-wheat flour

2 large eggs

1 tablespoon sugar

1 teaspoon grated orange zest

1 teaspoon canola or corn oil

....

Cooking spray

SAUCE

¼ cup light tub margarine

½ cup fresh orange juice (from about 2 medium oranges)

¼ cup orange liqueur or fresh orange juice

¼ cup sugar

1 teaspoon grated orange zest

....

1 cup fresh or frozen unsweetened raspberries, thawed if frozen

¼ cup brandy (optional)

In a medium mixing bowl, using an electric mixer on medium speed, beat together the milk, flour, eggs, sugar, 1 teaspoon orange zest, and the oil until well combined. Line a plate with paper towels.

Lightly spray an 8- or 10-inch skillet with cooking spray. Heat over medium heat. When the skillet is hot, remove from the heat. Spoon in ¼ cup crepe batter. Lift and tilt the skillet to spread the batter evenly. Return to the heat.

Cook the crepe for 3 to 4 minutes, or until the bottom is lightly browned. Turn over the crepe. Cook for about 20 seconds, or until lightly browned. Transfer the crepe to the paper towels. Repeat with the remaining batter, lightly spraying the skillet with cooking spray if necessary. You should have 8 or 9 crepes.

Fold each crepe in half. Fold in half again, forming a rounded triangle. Set aside.

Increase the heat to medium high. In a large skillet, stir together the margarine, orange juice, liqueur, and the remaining ¼ cup sugar and 1 teaspoon orange zest. Bring to a boil. Reduce the heat and simmer for 5 minutes, or until thickened, stirring occasionally.

Arrange the folded crepes in the sauce. Sprinkle the raspberries over the crepes. Simmer for 3 to 5 minutes, or until just heated through, spooning the sauce over the crepes and raspberries once or twice.

Meanwhile, in a small saucepan, heat the brandy if desired, until almost simmering. Carefully ignite it and pour it over the crepes. When the flames subside, swirl the skillet to distribute the brandy. Serve warm.

PER SERVING

Calories 165	Cholesterol 47 mg	DIETARY EXCHANGES:
Total Fat 4.5 g	Sodium 80 mg	1½ other carbohydrate
Saturated Fat 0.5 g	Carbohydrates 25 g	½ lean meat
Trans Fat 0.0 g	Fiber 2 g	½ fat
Polyunsaturated Fat 1.0 g	Sugars 15 g	
Monounsaturated Fat 2.0 g	Protein 5 g	

Apple-Raisin Sauce

Serves 6

Save lots of time, effort, and fat grams by serving this fruit sauce over fat-free vanilla ice cream or frozen yogurt instead of indulging in apple strudel à la mode. The sauce, which has no added sugar, is also a perfect topper for a slice of roast turkey or glazed ham.

3 **medium apples, peeled if desired, coarsely chopped**
2 **cups 100% apple juice**
¼ **cup raisins or dried cranberries**
1 **teaspoon ground cinnamon**
1 **tablespoon cornstarch**
2 **tablespoons cold water**

In a large saucepan, bring the apples, apple juice, raisins, and cinnamon to a boil over medium-high heat. Reduce the heat and simmer for 15 minutes, or until the apples are tender.

Meanwhile, put the cornstarch in a small bowl. Add the water, whisking to dissolve. Stir the cornstarch mixture into the cooked apple mixture. Cook for 1 to 2 minutes, or until thickened, stirring constantly.

Serve warm.

PER SERVING

Calories 96	Cholesterol 0 mg	DIETARY EXCHANGES:
Total Fat 0.0 g	Sodium 4 mg	1½ fruit
Saturated Fat 0.0 g	Carbohydrates 25 g	
Trans Fat 0.0 g	Fiber 2 g	
Polyunsaturated Fat 0.0 g	Sugars 19 g	
Monounsaturated Fat 0.0 g	Protein 1 g	

Bananas Foster Plus

Serves 4

Created in 1951 in Brennan's restaurant in New Orleans and named after a friend of the restaurant owner, this famous dessert has been lightened up and made more heart healthy with a pretty trio of caramelized fruit.

2 tablespoons light tub margarine

2 tablespoons plus 2 teaspoons light brown sugar

¼ teaspoon ground cinnamon

⅛ teaspoon ground nutmeg

2 medium bananas, cut into ½-inch slices

2 kiwifruit, peeled and cut into ½-inch slices

1 medium peach, peeled, or nectarine, peeled if desired, cut into ½-inch slices, or ½ cup canned sliced peaches in juice, drained

1 tablespoon dark rum or ¼ teaspoon rum extract

2 cups fat-free, sugar-free vanilla frozen yogurt or ice cream

In a medium skillet, melt the margarine over medium heat, swirling to coat the bottom.

Stir in the brown sugar, cinnamon, and nutmeg. Cook for 3 to 5 minutes, or until the sugar melts and the mixture is the desired consistency, stirring constantly.

Gently stir in the bananas, kiwifruit, and peach. Cook for 1 minute, or until heated through, gently stirring constantly.

Stir in the rum. Cook for 1 minute, gently stirring constantly.

Scoop the frozen yogurt into dessert bowls. Spoon the banana mixture over the yogurt.

PER SERVING

Calories 223	Cholesterol 3 mg	DIETARY EXCHANGES:
Total Fat 3.5 g	Sodium 104 mg	1½ fruit
Saturated Fat 0.5 g	Carbohydrates 45 g	1½ other carbohydrate
Trans Fat 0.0 g	Fiber 5 g	½ fat
Polyunsaturated Fat 0.5 g	Sugars 31 g	
Monounsaturated Fat 1.5 g	Protein 4 g	

Strawberries Romanoff

Serves 6

This dreamy dessert can also be served as a breakfast treat; just leave out the liqueur and sprinkle with crunchy whole-grain cereal. For flavor variety, try substituting other fruits and complementary liqueurs.

SAUCE

- 1 cup fat-free plain Greek yogurt
- ¼ cup firmly packed light brown sugar
- 2 tablespoons fruit-flavored liqueur, such as orange or strawberry (optional)
- 1 teaspoon vanilla extract
- ½ teaspoon ground cinnamon

. . . .

- 2 pints hulled strawberries, cut into bite-size pieces
- 2 tablespoons finely chopped pecans, dry-roasted

In a small bowl, whisk together the sauce ingredients until combined. Cover and refrigerate for at least 1 hour, or until slightly firm.

Spoon the berries into dessert dishes. Spoon the sauce over the berries. Sprinkle with the pecans.

PER SERVING

Calories 106	Cholesterol 2 mg	DIETARY EXCHANGES:
Total Fat 2.0 g	Sodium 17 mg	½ fruit
Saturated Fat 0.0 g	Carbohydrates 18 g	½ other carbohydrate
Trans Fat 0.0 g	Fiber 2 g	½ fat
Polyunsaturated Fat 0.5 g	Sugars 15 g	
Monounsaturated Fat 1.0 g	Protein 5 g	

Very Berry Sorbet

To freeze or not to freeze, that is the question. With this slightly tart dessert, both approaches yield unquestionably delicious results.

    1½ **cups frozen unsweetened blackberries, slightly thawed**
    2 **teaspoons water**
    1 **teaspoon frozen 100% orange juice concentrate, slightly thawed**
    1 **teaspoon brandy or cognac (optional)**
       Sprigs of fresh mint (optional)

In a food processor or blender, process all the ingredients except the mint until smooth.

If serving immediately, spoon into dessert bowls. Garnish with the mint sprigs. If serving later, spoon without the mint into an airtight freezer container and freeze. Let stand at room temperature for about 15 minutes before serving to soften.

PER SERVING

Calories 77	Cholesterol 0 mg	DIETARY EXCHANGES:
Total Fat 0.5 g	Sodium 1 mg	1½ fruit
Saturated Fat 0.0 g	Carbohydrates 19 g	
Trans Fat 0.0 g	Fiber 6 g	
Polyunsaturated Fat 0.5 g	Sugars 13 g	
Monounsaturated Fat 0.0 g	Protein 1 g	

Strawberry Margarita Ice

Serves 6

This frosty dessert takes its key ingredients from the ever-popular frozen margarita and is a perfectly refreshing treat on a hot summer's day. Enjoy it at your next barbecue after Southwestern Black Bean Spread (page 35) and Grilled Vegetable Quesadillas (page 230).

- 2 **cups fresh or frozen unsweetened strawberries, hulled if fresh, thawed if frozen**
- ½ **cup fresh orange juice**
- ¼ **cup fresh lime juice**
- ¼ **cup agave syrup**
- 1 **tablespoon tequila or fresh lime juice**
- 1 **tablespoon orange liqueur or fresh orange juice**

In a food processor or blender, process all the ingredients until smooth. Pour into a 9 x 5 x 3-inch loaf pan. Cover and freeze for 4 hours, or until firm but not frozen solid.

Meanwhile, put a large mixing bowl in the refrigerator to chill.

When the mixture is firm, break it into chunks and transfer them to the chilled bowl. Using an electric mixer, beat until smooth but not melted. Serve immediately or return the mixture to the loaf pan, cover, and freeze until serving time. To serve when frozen, using a spoon, scrape across the surface and mound the shavings in dessert dishes or margarita glasses.

....

COOK'S TIP: If you happen to leave the strawberry mixture in the freezer until it becomes frozen solid, let it stand at room temperature for 15 minutes. You'll then be able to break it into chunks and beat it as directed.

....

PER SERVING

Calories 81	Cholesterol 0 mg	DIETARY EXCHANGES:
Total Fat 0.0 g	Sodium 1 mg	1 other carbohydrate
Saturated Fat 0.0 g	Carbohydrates 19 g	
Trans Fat 0.0 g	Fiber 1 g	
Polyunsaturated Fat 0.0 g	Sugars 16 g	
Monounsaturated Fat 0.0 g	**Protein 1 g**	

HEALTHY SHOPPING STRATEGIES

To make good choices as you stock your pantry, it's important to take the time to know what you are buying. To find the best foods, compare product labels and key words on packaging. It's easy to identify the products that contain saturated fat, trans fat, and sodium, and to find others that you can substitute to help your heart. The labeling on packaged foods and the ingredients lists give you all the information you need to put together delicious meals that will help you manage your intake of unhealthy fats and lower your cholesterol.

READ NUTRITION FACTS PANELS

The U.S. Food and Drug Administration (FDA) requires that all U.S. food manufacturers put a nutrition label on their products. This label contains important information you should pay attention to when grocery shopping. By reading these food labels, you'll be able to easily identify how many calories and nutrients you'll be consuming by eating that particular food.

Check total calories per serving. Look at the serving size and determine how many servings you're really consuming. If you eat double the servings, you also double the calories and nutrients. Think about how eating the food will affect your calorie balance, keeping in mind that for a 2,000-calorie diet.

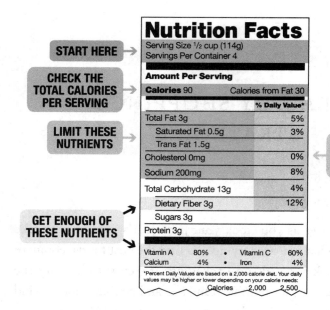

START HERE →

Nutrition Facts

Serving Size ½ cup (114g)
Servings Per Container 4

Amount Per Serving

CHECK THE TOTAL CALORIES PER SERVING →

Calories 90	Calories from Fat 30

	% Daily Value*

LIMIT THESE NUTRIENTS →

Total Fat 3g	5%
Saturated Fat 0.5g	3%
Trans Fat 1.5g	
Cholesterol 0mg	0%
Sodium 200mg	8%

← **Quick Guide to % DV 5% or less is low 20% or more is high**

Total Carbohydrate 13g	4%
Dietary Fiber 3g	12%
Sugars 3g	

Protein 3g

GET ENOUGH OF THESE NUTRIENTS

| Vitamin A | 80% | • | Vitamin C | 60% |
| Calcium | 4% | • | Iron | 4% |

*Percent Daily Values are based on a 2,000 calorie diet. Your daily values may be higher or lower depending on your calorie needs:
Calories 2,000 2,500

- 40 calories per serving is considered low;
- 100 calories per serving is considered moderate; and
- 400 calories or more per serving is considered high.

Limit certain nutrients. Take note of how much saturated fat, trans fat, and sodium are in each serving. Choose products that have lower amounts of each of these nutrients. Keep in mind that the American Heart Association recommends consuming no more than 1,500 mg of sodium a day for the greatest effect on blood pressure. So, for example, if a food has 800 mg per serving, then just by eating that one serving of that particular food you'll have consumed more than half of the association's recommended daily allowance.

Trace amounts of trans fats occur naturally in foods such as red meat and whole milk (even though the trans fat may be listed as zero on the label). However, by limiting red meat and choosing skinless poultry, oily fish, and nuts and using fat-free or low-fat dairy products, you can easily stay within the recommended limit for trans fat and saturated fat combined.

Understand % DV. The % DV section tells you the percentage of each nutrient in a single serving, in terms of the daily recommended amount. As a guide, if you want to consume less of a nutrient, such as saturated fat or sodium, choose foods with a lower % DV (5 percent or less is considered low). If you want to consume more of a nutrient, such as fiber, look for foods with a higher % DV (20 percent or more is considered high).

READ INGREDIENTS LISTS

When reading food labels, also look at the ingredients lists. Ingredients are listed in descending order, with the greatest amount first and the least amount last. When checking on saturated and trans fats in foods, watch for ingredients such as palm oil, palm kernel oil, and coconut oil. Be aware that the term "vegetable oil" can mean coconut, palm, or palm kernel oil, each of which is high in saturated fat. Look instead for products that list a specific polyunsaturated or monounsaturated vegetable oil, such as olive, canola, or corn oil.

Be aware of ingredients going by names other than the ones we expect. You might see sugar listed as the fourth ingredient in a product and think that's not so bad. But sugar can also be listed as high-fructose corn syrup or corn syrup, fructose, agave nectar, barley malt syrup, or dehydrated cane juice, to name just a few. Also, many different sodium compounds are added to foods. Watch for the words "soda" and "sodium" and the symbol "Na" on labels; these show that sodium compounds are present.

UNDERSTAND KEY WORDS ON FOOD PACKAGING

The U.S. Food and Drug Administration (USDA) has guidelines for the descriptors (see the table on the following page) that food manufacturers are allowed to put on their packages. Whether you're reducing your blood cholesterol level, watching your weight, or both, it pays to read these descriptors carefully.

KEY WORDS	PER SERVING
Fat-free	Less than 0.5 g fat
Low saturated fat	1 g or less
Low-fat	3 g or less
Reduced-fat	At least 25 percent less fat than the regular version
Light	Half the fat of the regular version
Low-cholesterol	20 mg or less, and 2 g or less of saturated fat
Low-sodium	140 mg sodium or less
Lean	Less than 10 g fat, 4.5 g or less saturated fat, and less than 95 mg cholesterol
Extra lean	Less than 5 g fat and less than 95 mg cholesterol

LOOK FOR THE HEART-CHECK MARK

The American Heart Association's Heart-Check mark on food packaging can help you easily and reliably identify foods that can be part of a heart-healthy diet. Foods bearing the iconic red heart with a white check mark meet specific nutrition requirements that limit saturated fat, trans fat, sodium, and added sugars, and promote consumption of beneficial nutrients. The nutrition requirements are food category–based and intended for healthy people over age two. People with special medical needs or dietary restrictions should follow the advice of their health professionals. To learn more about the Heart-Check mark and find a list of certified products, visit heartcheckmark.org.

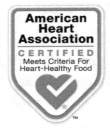

FIND INGREDIENT EQUIVALENTS

To make shopping easier, we have listed commonly used ingredients and their weight and volume equivalents. For example, if you see "1 cup chopped onion" in a recipe, you'll know that you need to have one large onion on hand to prepare that dish.

INGREDIENT	MEASUREMENT
Almonds	1 ounce = ¼ cup slivers
Apple	1 medium = ¾ cup chopped, 1 cup sliced
Basil, fresh	⅔ ounce = ½ cup, chopped, stems discarded
Bell pepper, any color	1 medium = 1 cup chopped or sliced
Carrot	1 medium = ⅓ to ½ cup chopped or sliced, ½ cup shredded
Celery	1 medium rib = ½ cup chopped or sliced
Cheese, hard, such as Parmesan	4 ounces = 1 cup grated 3½ ounces = 1 cup shredded
Cheese, semihard, such as Cheddar, mozzarella, or Swiss	4 ounces = 1 cup grated
Cheese, soft, such as blue, feta, or goat	1 ounce, crumbled = ¼ cup
Cucumber	1 medium = 1 cup sliced
Lemon juice	1 medium = 3 tablespoons
Lemon zest	1 medium = 2 to 3 teaspoons
Lime juice	1 medium = 1½ to 2 tablespoons
Lime zest	1 medium = 1 teaspoon
Mushrooms (button)	1 pound = 5 cups sliced or 6 cups chopped

INGREDIENT	MEASUREMENT
Onions, green	8 to 9 medium = 1 cup sliced (green and white parts)
Onions, white or yellow	1 large = 1 cup chopped 1 medium = 2/3 cup chopped 1 small = 1/3 cup chopped
Orange juice	1 medium = 1/3 to 1/2 cup
Orange zest	1 medium = 1 1/2 to 2 tablespoons
Strawberries	1 pint = 2 cups sliced or chopped
Tomatoes	2 large, 3 medium, or 4 small = 1 1/2 to 2 cups chopped
Walnuts	1 ounce = 1/4 cup chopped

HEALTHY COOKING STRATEGIES

As you prepare the recipes in this book, your time in the kitchen will be well spent. With each satisfying meal, you will be helping your heart. To create these healthy dishes, we rely on certain principles that allow us to cut back on saturated fat, trans fat, added sugar, and sodium without losing flavor and appeal. You can apply the same techniques to all the foods you cook at home. Simply start out with wholesome ingredients and then use one of the following techniques to create a delicious and nutritious meal.

CHOOSE HIGH-FLAVOR, LOW-FAT PREPARATIONS

You can avoid a great deal of saturated fat by using several healthy cooking techniques instead of deep-fat frying or panfrying. You'll find that these cooking methods result in dishes that are just as tasty as their higher-saturated-fat counterparts.

As you prepare meals, use nonstick cookware, cooking spray, or a bit of unsaturated oil instead of butter or margarine to keep foods from sticking as they cook. You can follow this heart-healthy practice with most recipes and most of the cooking techniques below, which are the ones you'll see most frequently in this cookbook.

BRAISING

Braising involves layering flavors in a heavy pot that's tightly covered. It often begins with a foundation of caramelized poultry or meat to which herbs, aromatics, and vegetables are added before the whole dish is simmered in a small amount of fragrant liquid such as wine, beer, broth, vinegar, or fruit juice. Because herbs and aromatics are an important element in braising, they provide enough flavoring that little salt—if any—is needed. Braising is also a good method for cooking firm vegetables.

STEWING

Stewing is similar to braising except that the food is covered by the cooking liquid. If you like to cook one-dish meals, then stewing is an ideal technique for you. Fish, poultry, beans, or meat can easily be combined with vegetables in a pot to make dinner. A tight-fitting cover on the stew pot minimizes evaporation, and the condensation formed inside acts as a self-basting process to keep the food moist while locking in the nutrients. Stewing is good for some fresh fruits, such as peaches, plums, apples, pears, and cherries, and for dried fruits.

GRILLING

Grilling is an easy way to cook quick, healthy meals. The grilled foods cook fast so they retain their moisture and excess unhealthy fats drip away into the grill. The intense, direct heat provides a crisp, browned crust and a moist, tender interior, and the quick cooking lets you get dinner on the table in short order. You can use the surface of the grill to cook both your entrée and side dishes. Although poultry and lean meats are popular grilling choices, you can also use this healthy cooking technique to incorporate a variety of food groups into your meals, including seafood, vegetables, and fruit. Grilling brings out such unique, natural sweet flavors that it's a perfect opportunity to try foods you may not have eaten before. Marinades, rubs, and sauces are good flavor enhancers for grilled foods. Just be sure to look for those that are low in sodium, saturated and trans fats, and added sugar.

BROILING

Think of broiling simply as upside-down grilling with the food on the bottom and the flame or heating element on top. The speed and simplicity of broiling—and the fact that ovens come equipped with a built-in broiler—make it a convenient and simple way to prepare healthy meals. Just about anything that you can grill can be broiled, including many nutritious foods, such as seafood, vegetables, and even fruit. The intense, direct heat cooks food fast and caramelizes it, giving it a distinctive flavor. Trim all visible fat before grilling or broiling; doing so will not only cut down on the amount of "bad" fat but also help prevent flare-ups. One important note about broiling: If your recipe says, for example, to broil about 4 inches from the heat, that means 4 inches from the heat element to the top of the food you are broiling, not to the top of the broiling rack.

MICROWAVING

Microwave cooking uses moist heat, making it an especially healthy way to prepare vegetables, fruits, and fish. That's because very little liquid is needed, so nutrients are retained. You can cook such a variety of healthy meals in a hurry using the microwave that you may never heat up your oven again. How do microwaves cook food so fast? Contrary to the popular misconception, microwaves don't cook food from the inside out. Rather, they penetrate the food from every direction so food cooks much faster than it would in a traditional oven. Another benefit of microwave cooking is that foods don't stick, and cleanup is easy. To avoid both overcooking and undercooking meat and poultry, use a meat thermometer to check doneness. Remove the meat or poultry from the oven before inserting the instant-read thermometer. Insert the thermometer into the center, or thickest part, of the meat, making sure the thermometer doesn't touch bone or fat.

POACHING

Poaching is a simple way to prepare meals, especially delicate foods such as eggs, seafood, and fruit. Poaching brings water or a flavorful poaching liquid, such as wine, broth, fruit juice, or tea, to a boil and then gently simmers the food until done, which helps retain the food's shape and moisture. Although the liquid does come to a boil at first, poaching shouldn't be confused with cooking by boiling. And once the food is poached, the liquid often becomes a tasty base for a sauce, which means you retain all the food's vitamins and minerals. Poaching is a great cooking method for infusing chicken breasts with tons of flavor while keeping them moist and tender.

STEAMING

Steaming is one of the best ways to retain a food's color and preserve its nutrients. By varying the steaming liquid and adding spices and aromatics, you can infuse steamed dishes with delicate flavor; for more intense flavor, add aromatics such as garlic and onion to the food itself or pair the food with a delicious sauce. Because steam transfers heat to food more efficiently than either boiling water or hot air, steaming is one of the quickest cooking techniques. Steaming is ideal for vegetables. You can keep it super simple by adding any fresh vegetable to a steamer basket. With steaming, you can incorporate more grains into your diet; this technique makes them light and fluffy. Most steaming is done by placing the food in a bamboo steamer or collapsible metal or silicone basket suspended over simmering liquid; the food is cooked by gentle hot vapor. Food cooked *en papillote,* or enclosed in a packet of cooking parchment or aluminum foil and cooked in the oven, is also a form of steaming that uses the foods' own juices to cook. This method makes portion control and cleanup a snap.

STIR-FRYING

Stir-frying is a healthy, quick, cost-conscious, and efficient cooking method. Within minutes, a nutritious meal can be put together complete with plenty of vegetables and a protein such as fish, poultry, meat, tofu, or lentils. Stir-fried dishes commonly include more than one type of vegetable, allowing for a variety of nutrients and the opportunity to include different produce in your eating plan. Stir-frying requires a minimum of hot oil, and this fast, high-heat method of cooking seals in the natural juices of seafood and meats and preserves the nutrients, texture, and color of vegetables. Stir-frying is typically done in a wok, although a large skillet also works well. The high temperature and the constant movement of the food keep it from sticking and burning. Once you actually start stir-frying, everything moves quickly, so slice or dice each ingredient into uniform pieces (for more even cooking) and prepare any sauces before you begin.

ROASTING

Roasting uses the dry heat of an oven and is usually done without a cover and at higher heat. This technique is best for tender foods and larger cuts of meat, poultry, and fish, such as whole chickens or turkeys, pork or beef tenderloin, whole fish, or thick fish fillets. When roasting meat, discard the visible fat and place the meat on a rack in a roasting pan to prevent the meat from sitting in its fat drippings. If needed, baste it with fat-free liquids, such as wine, fruit juice, or fat-free, low-sodium broth. Plan on removing the meat from the oven 15 to 20 minutes before serving. Letting the meat "rest" retains the juices and makes it easier to carve. For whole birds, discard as much fat as you can before roasting, but leave the skin on until the poultry is cooked. Discard the skin before serving the poultry. Roasting also works well for a number of fruits, such as peaches and bananas, and vegetables from asparagus to zucchini, but not green, leafy vegetables.

Baking uses the dry heat of an oven, may or may not use a cover, and usually involves somewhat lower heat. The gentle heat of the oven not only melds flavors but can also provide crisp textures. This technique is ideal for smaller pieces of meat, chicken breasts, or fish fillets. Baking can tenderize large vegetables, such as squash. It also can mimic the crisp exteriors of fried foods such as baked sweet potato french fries and is an ideal technique for classic family favorites, such as meat loaf and spinach.

HEALTHY COOKING TIPS

Here are some tips for heart-smart cooking as well as ways to help trim calories and unhealthy nutrients from your home-cooked dishes—without trimming taste.

SEAFOOD, POULTRY, AND MEATS

- Try grilling or broiling fish, either directly on the grill or broiler pan or wrapped in aluminum foil. Using a few herbs and some citrus juice as seasoning will let you enjoy the wonderful flavor of the fish itself instead of tasting the batter and the frying oil.
- Remove all visible fat before cooking meat or poultry.
- If you're using leftover marinade for basting or in a sauce, take precautions: Be sure to boil the marinade for at least 5 minutes before using it to kill any harmful bacteria that the raw food may have transmitted.
- Before cooking most chicken dishes, discard the skin and all visible fat. Be sure to scrub the cutting surface and utensils well with hot, sudsy water after preparing poultry for cooking. If you're roasting a chicken, leave the skin on to prevent the chicken from drying out. Discard the skin before serving the chicken.

- Baste meats and poultry with low-sodium broth, wine, or fruit juice instead of melted butter or other liquids high in saturated fat.
- Buy turkeys that are not self-basting. Many self-basting turkeys are high in saturated fat and sodium.

VEGETABLES

- To retain natural juices, wrap food in aluminum foil before grilling or baking. Also try wrapping food in edible pouches made of steamed lettuce or cabbage leaves.
- Cook most vegetables just long enough to make them tender-crisp. Overcooked vegetables lose both flavor and important nutrients. With more natural flavor, there's less temptation to use butter or rich sauces.
- Cut down on saturated fats by using more vegetables and less poultry, seafood, or meat in soups, stews, and casseroles. Finely chopped vegetables and whole grains also are great for stretching ground poultry or meat.
- When you make stuffing, substitute chopped vegetables for some of the bread.

SOUPS, SAUCES, AND GRAVIES

- After making soups and sauces, refrigerate them and skim the hardened fat off the top.
- Instead of using a roux (butter-flour mixture) to thicken soups, stews, or sauces, use pureed cooked vegetables or a tablespoon of cornstarch or flour blended with a cup of room-temperature fat-free, low-sodium broth or water. Add the blended liquid and simmer until the dish thickens.

- Substitute herbs, spices, and salt-free seasonings for salt as you cook and at the table.
- Substitute onion or garlic flakes or powder for onion or garlic salt.
- Add a bit of lemon juice to the water in which you cook pasta, and eliminate the salt.
- Reduce or omit salt in baking recipes that don't use yeast.
- Use wheat germ, bran, whole-wheat unseasoned bread crumbs or panko, or matzo meal in place of buttered crumbs as toppings.
- Instead of croutons, fried bacon, or fried onion rings in salads and casseroles, try nuts or water chestnuts for added crunch.

ADAPT YOUR OWN RECIPES

If you're afraid you'll have to give up your favorite recipes to eat heart-healthy, don't worry. You can still enjoy most of your favorite dishes simply by making a few easy substitutions to cut back on saturated and trans fats, added sugar, and sodium.

WHEN YOUR RECIPE CALLS FOR	USE INSTEAD
Regular broth or bouillon	Low-sodium broths, either homemade or commercially prepared; low-sodium bouillon granules or cubes, reconstituted according to package directions (be sure to select products made without partially hydrogenated oils).
Butter or shortening	When possible, use fat-free spray margarine or fat-free or light tub margarine made from vegetable oil. Some recipes do not adapt as well as others to substituting fats. Try different products until you find one that works for your recipe and choose the product that is lowest in saturated and trans fats by selecting products made without partially hydrogenated oils.

WHEN YOUR RECIPE CALLS FOR	USE INSTEAD
Butter for sautéing	Vegetable oil or cooking spray; fat-free, low-sodium broth; wine; fruit or vegetable juice.
Cream	Low-fat or fat-free options for half-and-half; nondairy creamer; evaporated milk.
Evaporated milk	Low-fat or fat-free evaporated milk.
Flavored salts, such as onion salt, garlic salt, and celery salt	Onion powder, garlic powder, celery seeds or flakes. Use about one-fourth the amount of flavored salt indicated in the recipe.
Ice cream	Fat-free, low-fat, or light ice cream; fat-free or low-fat frozen yogurt; sorbet; sherbet; gelato.
Oil in baking	Unsweetened applesauce.
Table salt	No-salt-added seasoning blends.
Tomato juice	No-salt-added tomato juice.
Tomato sauce	No-salt-added tomato sauce; 6-ounce can of no-salt-added tomato paste diluted with 1 can of water.
Unsweetened baking chocolate	3 tablespoons cocoa powder plus 1 tablespoon polyunsaturated oil or unsaturated tub margarine for every 1-ounce square of chocolate.
Whipping cream	Fat-free whipped topping (be sure to select a product made without partially hydrogenated oils); fat-free evaporated milk (thoroughly chilled before whipping).
Whole milk	Low-fat or fat-free milk.

STOCK A HEART-HEALTHY PANTRY

Keeping healthy staples on hand makes cooking healthy meals at home easier and more convenient. Don't let the long list discourage you; most of these items aren't perishable or have a fairly long shelf life so you can acquire them over time to build up your pantry. If you keep some healthy basics in each category, you'll have more options for cooking nutritious meals at home. In fact, you'll be able to prepare most of the recipes in this book with the ingredients waiting in your well-stocked refrigerator, freezer, and pantry; for many other dishes, you'll need only a few additional items from the store.

garlic

gingerroot

lemons

limes

onions

oranges

shallots

various chiles

eggs

egg substitute

fat-free or low-fat feta cheese

fat-free half-and-half

fat-free milk

fat-free plain Greek yogurt

fat-free plain yogurt

fat-free ricotta cheese

fat-free sour cream

light mayonnaise

light tub margarine

low-fat buttermilk

low-fat Cheddar cheese

low-fat mozzarella cheese

Parmesan cheese, shaved, shredded, or grated

Queso fresco or farmer cheese

assorted fruits and berries

assorted vegetables without added sauces

brown rice

chicken breasts

extra-lean ground beef

fish fillets

ground skinless chicken breast

ground skinless turkey breast

lean steaks and chops

seitan

soy crumbles

tofu

turkey bacon

FOR THE PANTRY (NON-PERISHABLES)

RICES (CHOOSE UNSEASONED)

Arborio rice

instant and/or regular brown rice

BEANS AND LEGUMES

dried beans, peas, and lentils

no-salt-added canned black beans

no-salt-added canned cannellini beans

no-salt-added canned chickpeas

no-salt-added canned kidney beans

no-salt-added canned navy beans

PASTAS AND GRAINS

assorted whole-grain and enriched pastas, including
lasagna noodles

barley

corn tortillas

farro

instant, or fine-grain, bulgur

regular and quick-cooking oatmeal

quinoa

whole-wheat couscous

dry-packed sun-dried tomatoes

no-salt-added diced, stewed, crushed, and whole
tomatoes

no-salt-added tomato paste

no-salt-added tomato sauce

spaghetti sauce (lowest sodium available)

DRY GOODS

active dry yeast

baking powder

baking soda

cornmeal

cornstarch

flour: all-purpose, whole-wheat, white whole-
wheat, and whole-wheat pastry

green tea bags

plain dry bread crumbs (lowest sodium available)

salt-free instant bouillon: chicken and beef

sugar: granulated, light brown, dark brown, and
confectioners'

whole-wheat panko (Japanese-style bread crumbs)

CANNED AND BOTTLED PRODUCTS

100% fruit juices

boneless, skinless salmon canned or in pouches
(lowest sodium available)

canned very low sodium tuna, packed in water

canned water chestnuts

fat-free, low-sodium broths: chicken, beef, and/or
vegetable

fruits canned in water with no sugar added when
possible or in their own juice

garlic: minced, chopped, or whole cloves

gingerroot, minced

green chiles

kalamata olives

light beer

low-sodium soups

no-salt-added canned vegetables

red wine (regular or nonalcoholic)

roasted red bell peppers

sherry (not cooking sherry)

unsweetened applesauce

white wine (regular or nonalcoholic)

COOKING OILS

canola or corn oil

cooking sprays

olive oil

peanut oil

toasted sesame oil

MISCELLANEOUS

all-fruit spreads

dried fruits, including raisins, cranberries, apricots, and plums (choose those with the least added sugar)

honey

low-sodium peanut butter

molasses

pure maple syrup

seeds, including sesame, anise, caraway, fennel, and pumpkin (unsalted)

unsalted nuts, including almonds, walnuts, peanuts, pecans, and pine nuts

chipotle peppers canned in adobo sauce

hot chili oil

mustards

no-salt-added ketchup

red hot-pepper sauce

soy sauce

Thai sweet chile sauce

vinegars, including cider, balsamic, red wine, white
wine, and plain rice

Worcestershire sauce

SPICES AND SEASONINGS

black pepper

cayenne

chili powder

crushed red pepper flakes

curry powder

dried herbs, including oregano, basil, thyme,
rosemary, dillweed, parsley, sage, bay leaves,
and saffron

dry mustard

garlic powder

ground spices, including cinnamon, ginger, nutmeg,
allspice, cumin, coriander, paprika, smoked
paprika, and turmeric

onion powder

salt

salt-free seasoning blends, including all-purpose,
Creole or Cajun, Italian, and lemon pepper

vanilla extract

HEALTHY DINING OUT STRATEGIES

If you're like many other Americans, you don't always make dinner but rather you make reservations or you head out for a quick bite more than half the time. Instead of feeling guilty and worrying about how restaurant food will affect your heart, learn how to eat out with your heart in mind. What are you in the mood for today? Whether you eat out a lot or only once in a while, these tips will help you make better choices of what to eat.

KNOW BEFORE YOU GO

- Visit websites of fast-food and casual dining restaurants and print out the nutritional information for their meal choices. Keep the printouts where you can refer to them when you make food selections.
- Avoid all-you-can-eat buffets. It's very hard not to overeat.

ORDER WITH YOUR HEART IN MIND

- In general, try to eat a small amount of meat and lots of vegetables.
- Request smaller portions or plan to share entrées. Ask for a to-go box and plan to take home a part of your meal.
- Select foods with less cheese and sauce, or ask for those extras on the side. That way you can control how much of them you eat.

- When you order side dishes, ask the kitchen to omit any sauces, margarine, or butter.
- Feel free to ask about ingredients or how a dish is prepared. Don't hesitate to request substitutions or a specially prepared dish. Many chefs are eager to please.
- Choose broiled, baked, grilled, steamed, or poached entrées over the high-fat fried ones.
- Order potatoes baked, boiled, or roasted—not fried. Then leave off the butter and margarine. Try fat-free or low-fat sour cream, pepper, and chives instead. Salsa is also an excellent potato topper.
- Order salad dressings on the side so you can control your portions. Better yet, try a squeeze of lemon instead of rich dressings.
- Ask for whole-grain breads and rolls when available. Another good choice is melba toast. Use olive oil or soft margarine instead of butter or stick margarine.
- Drink water, fat-free or low-fat milk, or unsweetened coffee or tea instead of sugar-laden soda and juice drinks.
- For dessert, choose something light, such as fresh fruit or sorbet.

SMART STRATEGIES BY CUISINE

No matter where you are, use your head to make wise choices for your heart. Here are specific strategies geared to several popular restaurant types.

FAST FOOD

- Pass up the "value size" meal options, and avoid double meat. That's almost certainly much more than the recommended serving size of 2 to 3 ounces.

- Order salad for your main dish, and choose grilled or broiled chicken breast options without breading.
- Avoid mayonnaise and other high-calorie dressings and sauces. Onions, lettuce, and tomato add flavor without saturated fat or sodium. Use pickles and ketchup sparingly because of their high sodium content.
- Have a side salad instead of the usual french fries.
- Skip the bacon on your sandwich or salad.

ASIAN

- Choose a steamed or poached main dish or try a stir-fried chicken or seafood and vegetable dish.
- Ask the chef to use a minimal amount of oil and leave out the soy sauce, MSG, and salt.
- Choose entrées with lots of vegetables.
- Instead of tempura-style vegetables, ask for steamed or stir-fried vegetables.
- Ask for brown rice instead of white and steamed instead of fried.
- Avoid the crisp fried noodles usually served as an appetizer.

ITALIAN

- Opt for pasta with a small amount of olive oil or with marinara or marsala sauce instead of pasta with a cream sauce, such as Alfredo.
- Try a seafood selection or meatless pasta in place of an entrée with sausage or meatballs.
- If you order pizza, choose one with a thin crust. Opt for toppings such as spinach, mushrooms, broccoli, and roasted peppers instead of sausage or pepperoni.
- Ask for plain Italian bread instead of buttery garlic bread.

- Choose spicy grilled chicken or fish instead of a fried entrée.
- Ask your waiter to bring soft corn tortillas instead of the fried tortilla chips usually served as an appetizer.
- Choose corn tortillas rather than flour tortillas, which are usually high in sodium and may contain lard.
- Use salsa, pico de gallo, cilantro, and jalapeños for added flavor.
- If your entrée comes with sour cream, ask if fat-free or low-fat is available. If not, ask the kitchen to leave it off.
- Ask for a tomato-based sauce, such as ranchero, instead of a creamy or cheesy sauce, such as sour cream or queso.
- If you order a taco salad, don't eat the fried shell.

THE SCIENCE BEHIND
THE RECOMMENDATIONS

What happens in your body that turns foods that are supposed to help nourish into a potential threat instead? Here's a brief explanation of how the cholesterol in your body affects the well-being of your heart. This science forms the basis for the American Heart Association recommendations on how to eat better for better health.

HOW CHOLESTEROL AFFECTS YOUR HEART

Your body needs some cholesterol—a waxy fatlike substance—to strengthen cell walls and for other body functions, such as producing hormones. Your blood carries cholesterol and other fats through your body in distinct particles called *lipoproteins*. (Because lipids, or fats, do not mix with water, the body wraps them in protein to move them through the bloodstream.) Three types of lipoprotein make up the major part of your total blood cholesterol measurement: low-density lipoprotein (LDL), high-density lipoprotein (HDL), and very-low-density lipoprotein (VLDL).

A simple blood test will determine your cholesterol levels in milligrams per deciliter of blood (mg/dl). Your total cholesterol report is among numerous factors your doctor can use to predict your lifetime or 10-year risk for a heart attack or stroke.

A complete fasting lipoprotein profile will show the following:

TOTAL BLOOD CHOLESTEROL

Your total cholesterol score is calculated using the following equation: HDL + LDL + 20 percent of your triglyceride level. A total cholesterol score of less than 180 mg/dl is considered optimal.

HIGH-DENSITY LIPOPROTEIN (HDL)

HDL cholesterol is considered the "good" cholesterol because it helps remove the LDL cholesterol from the arteries. Experts believe that HDL acts as a scavenger, carrying LDL cholesterol away from the arteries and back to the liver, where it is broken down and passed from the body. A healthy level of HDL cholesterol may also protect against heart attack and stroke, while low levels of HDL cholesterol have been shown to increase the risk of heart disease and stroke.

LOW-DENSITY LIPOPROTEIN (LDL)

Low-density lipoproteins carry cholesterol to the inner walls of the arteries, where it can collect and contribute to the buildup of plaque. That process is called *atherosclerosis*. Plaque buildup narrows the artery walls and reduces the flow of blood. If a plaque ruptures, it triggers a blood clot to form. If the clot forms where the plaque is, it can block blood flow or break off and travel to another part of the body. If blood flow to an artery that feeds the heart is blocked, it causes a heart attack. If the blockage occurs in an artery that feeds the brain, it causes a stroke. Another condition called peripheral artery disease can develop when plaque buildup narrows an artery supplying blood to the legs. A low LDL cholesterol level is considered good for your heart health. However, your LDL number should no longer be the main factor in determining treatment to prevent a heart attack or stroke. For people taking statins, it is no longer necessary to get the LDL cholesterol number down to a specific target.

Triglycerides are another type of fat, and they're used to store excess energy from your diet. High levels of triglycerides in the blood are associated with atherosclerosis. Elevated triglycerides can be caused by being overweight or obese, physical inactivity, cigarette smoking, excess alcohol consumption, and a diet very high in carbohydrates (more than 60 percent of total calories).

EVOLVING SCIENCE

The American Heart Association released new cholesterol guidelines in November 2013. These guidelines no longer recommend people aim for a target cholesterol level but instead offer options based on an individual's risk of a heart attack or stroke; this risk can be determined through a new risk assessment calculator for healthcare professionals. Talk to your healthcare professional about what's best for you. Because science evolves, visit heart.org for more information on the latest findings.

RISK FACTORS FOR HEART DISEASE AND STROKE

Several conditions in addition to high blood cholesterol levels contribute to the risk for heart disease and stroke. Some are factors that cannot be changed. Others result from a combination of your habits and how your body reacts to those habits, and these are the factors you can change to reduce your risk.

RISK FACTORS YOU *CANNOT* CHANGE

Family History. The tendency toward heart disease seems to run in families. Children of parents with heart disease are more likely to develop it themselves, particularly if heart disease was a cause of premature death in the parents or grandparents. Race is also a factor. Compared with Caucasians, African-Americans develop high blood pressure earlier in life, and their average blood pressures are much higher. As a result, their risk of heart disease is greater.

Gender and Increasing Age. Earlier in life, men have a greater risk of heart attack than women. Men tend to have higher levels of LDL cholesterol and lower levels of HDL cholesterol than women. However, women's death rate from heart disease increases after menopause. Most people who die of a heart attack are age 65 or older. At older ages, women who have heart attacks are twice as likely as men to die within a few weeks of an attack.

RISK FACTORS YOU CAN CHANGE

High Blood Cholesterol. If you have high blood cholesterol, you can take steps to reduce it through diet and exercise and medication, if needed. For detailed information on how blood cholesterol affects your heart, see Appendix D, page 343.

High Blood Pressure. High blood pressure has no symptoms, which is why it's often called the silent killer. High blood pressure increases the risk of stroke, heart attack, kidney failure, and congestive heart failure. Have your blood pressure checked regularly. A blood pressure reading of 140/90 millimeters of mercury (mm Hg) or above is considered high and is referred to as hypertension. A blood pressure reading of 120/80 to 139/89 is considered prehypertension. Lifestyle changes such as eating a healthy diet, limiting sodium intake, being physically active, losing weight, and quitting smoking can help prevent or postpone the onset of high blood pressure. Your doctor can help you control existing high blood pressure through these same lifestyle changes and medication, if needed.

Physical Inactivity. Physical inactivity is another major risk factor for heart disease. Regular exercise can help control levels of harmful LDL cholesterol, raise levels of helpful HDL cholesterol, and lower blood pressure in some people. Lack of physical activity also increases the likelihood of being overweight or obese. Being physically active is an important part of lowering your risk for heart disease.

Overweight and Obesity. In addition to being considered a disease itself, obesity also is a risk factor for heart attack, congestive heart failure, sudden cardiac death, and angina, or chest pain. It puts added strain on the heart, which can lead to other serious conditions, such as weakened heart muscle and irregular heart rhythms. Being overweight or obese can lead to high blood pressure, increased LDL cholesterol, decreased HDL cholesterol, and increased triglyceride levels—and the risk of developing diabetes is greater as well. For more information, see "Manage Your Weight," page 21.

Smoking. A smoker's risk of coronary heart disease is two to three times that of a nonsmoker. Your risk of heart disease also increases if you breathe in secondhand smoke at home or at work. When you stop smoking, no matter how long or how much you have smoked, your risk of heart disease drops rapidly. Your risk for coronary heart disease, stroke, and peripheral vascular disease is reduced, and within one to two years after you quit, your risk of coronary heart disease is reduced substantially.

Diabetes. The 21 million Americans who have physician-diagnosed diabetes are major candidates for heart disease and stroke. Because the risk factors of having diabetes and being overweight often go hand in hand, it's especially important for diabetic patients to watch their diet, stay active, and maintain a healthy weight. You can reduce your risk of developing diabetes, or if you have diabetes, you can help control it by adopting the same recommendations that are good for your heart: Eat a healthy diet, be physically active, lose weight if needed, manage your blood pressure, stop smoking, and monitor and control your blood glucose levels.

Metabolic Syndrome. The term metabolic syndrome refers to a combination of any three or more of the following risk factors: a waist measurement greater than 40 inches for men and greater than 35 inches for women; a triglyceride level of 150 mg/dL and higher; HDL less than 40 mg/dL for men and less than 50 mg/dL for women; systolic blood pressure of 130 mm Hg or higher, or diastolic blood pressure of 85 mm Hg or higher; and a fasting glucose reading of 100 mg/dL or higher. With metabolic syndrome, the risk of heart disease that comes with high blood cholesterol is even greater.

WARNING SIGNS FOR HEART ATTACK AND STROKE

When you see the signs of a possible heart attack or stroke, every second counts. If you or someone near you experiences any of the symptoms listed below, act immediately and call 9-1-1.

HEART ATTACK WARNING SIGNS

- **Chest discomfort.** Most heart attacks involve discomfort in the center of the chest that lasts more than a few minutes, or that goes away and comes back. It can feel like uncomfortable pressure, squeezing, fullness, or pain.
- **Discomfort in other areas of the upper body.** Symptoms can include pain or discomfort in one or both arms, the back, neck, jaw, or stomach.
- **Shortness of breath.** This may occur with or without chest discomfort.
- **Other signs.** These may include breaking out in a cold sweat, nausea, or lightheadedness.

For both men and women, the most common heart attack symptom is chest pain or discomfort. However, women are somewhat more likely than men to experience some of the other common symptoms, particularly shortness of breath, nausea/vomiting, and back or jaw pain.

STROKE WARNING SIGNS

- Sudden numbness or weakness of the face, arm, or leg, especially on one side of the body
- Sudden confusion or trouble speaking or understanding
- Sudden trouble seeing in one or both eyes
- Sudden trouble walking, dizziness, loss of balance or coordination
- Sudden, severe headache with no known cause

F.A.S.T. is an easy way to remember how to recognize a stroke and what to do. Spot a stroke FAST. **F**ace drooping. **A**rm weakness. **S**peech difficulty. **T**ime to call 9-1-1.

index

A

almond flour
cook's tip on, 305
Maple-Blueberry Bars, 304–5
almonds
Crunchy-Crusted Salmon, 120–21
Trail Mix with Cocoa-Dusted Almonds, 38
Trout Amandine with Orange-Dijon Sauce, 132–33
appetizers and snacks
Banana Mini Snack Cakes, 45
Canapés with Roasted Garlic, Artichoke, and Chèvre Spread, 41
Creamy Caper Dip, 30
Fresh Basil and Kalamata Hummus, 34
Kale-and-Ham-Stuffed Cremini Mushrooms, 44
Nectarine-Plum Chutney, 39
Orange-Ginger Chicken Skewers, 40
Orange-Strawberry Froth, 47
Pineapple Shake, 48
Roasted Red Bell Pepper Dip, 31
Sangría-Style Pomegranate Coolers, 46
Smoked Salmon Dip with Cucumber and Herbs, 32
Southwestern Black Bean Spread, 35
Spiced Apple Cider, 49
Sweet-Spice Vanilla Dip with Dried Plums and Pecans, 33
Tomato Bursts, 37
Trail Mix with Cocoa-Dusted Almonds, 38

Zesty Potato Skins, 42–43
Zucchini Spread, 36
apple
Apple-Lemon Carrots, 255
Apple-Raisin Sauce, 314
Apple-Rhubarb Crisp, 298–99
coring, cook's tip on, 298
Puffed Pancake with Apple-Cranberry Sauce, 288–89
Skillet Pork Chops with Cinnamon-Apple Salsa, 209
Apple Cider, Spiced, 49
artichokes
Artichoke-Rotini Salad with Chicken, 92
Canapés with Roasted Garlic, Artichoke, and Chèvre Spread, 41
Creamy Artichoke Dressing, 97
Eggplant Parmigiana, 234–35
Grilled Cod with Artichoke-Horseradish Sauce, 114–15
Rosemary-Artichoke Frittata, 240–41
Slow-Cooker Tuscan Chicken, 162
asparagus
Asparagus with Dill and Pine Nuts, 250
Chilled Asparagus Soup, 58–59
cook's tip on, 59
Grilled Pizza with Grilled Vegetables, 212–13
avocados
cook's tip on, 35
Southwestern Black Bean Spread, 35
Tomatillo-Avocado Dressing, 101

B

Banana Mini Snack Cakes, 45
Bananas Foster Plus, 315
barley
    Carrot and Barley Pilaf, 254
    Chunky Barley Soup, 54
basil
    Broiled Salmon with Olive Pesto,
        122
    Fresh Basil and Kalamata
        Hummus, 34
    Mediterranean Strata, 245
    Thai, cook's tip on, 167
    Thai Chicken with Basil and
        Vegetables, 166–67
    Turkey Patties with Fresh
        Basil-Mushroom Sauce,
        178
beans
    Brunswick Stew, 163
    Bunless Beef-and-Bean Burgers,
        202
    Chili, 200–1
    Edamame Stir-Fry, 244
    Fiesta Black Bean Nachos, 232
    Fresh Basil and Kalamata
        Hummus, 34
    Greek Chopped Salad, 93
    Pasta e Fagioli, 214–15
    Pasta with Fresh Vegetable Sauce,
        220–21
    Rustic Tomato Soup, 66–67
    Southwestern Black Bean
        Spread, 35
    Spicy Chickpea and Chayote
        Soup, 68
    Spinach and Black Bean
        Enchiladas, 233
    Taco Salad, 94–95

Triple-Pepper and White Bean
    Soup with Rotini, 69
see also edamame; green beans;
    legumes
beef
    Balsamic Braised Beef with Exotic
        Mushrooms, 188
    Beef Tenderloin Roast, 180–81
    Bulgur and Ground Beef
        Casserole, 191
    Bunless Beef-and-Bean Burgers, 202
    Chili, 200–1
    Grilled Sirloin Steak with
        Chimichurri Sauce, 184–85
    Grilled Teriyaki Sirloin, 182–83
    Meatballs Hawaiian, 196–97
    Meat Loaf with Apricot Glaze,
        192–93
    Sirloin Steak with Portobello
        Mushrooms, 189
    Slow-Cooker Pepper Steak, 190
    Southwestern Beef Pita Tacos,
        198–99
    Spiced Shish Kebabs with
        Horseradish Cream, 186–87
    steak cuts, cook's tip on, 185
    Stuffed Cabbage Rolls, 194–95
    Taco Salad, 94–95
beets
    Beets in Orange Sauce, 248–49
    fresh, cook's tip on, 249
bell peppers
    Artichoke-Rotini Salad with
        Chicken, 92
    Bulgur and Butternut Squash, 228
    Cajun Chicken Pasta, 165
    Chicken and Veggie Bake, 169
    Chicken Fajitas, 154–55
    Chicken Southwestern, 156–57

352

Edamame Stir-Fry, 244
Fish Fillets with Broiled-Veggie
    Rice, 106–7
Greek-Style Stewed Chicken, 168
Grilled Pizza with Grilled
    Vegetables, 212–13
Grilled Vegetable Quesadillas,
    230–31
Hearty Fish Chowder, 108–9
Macaroni Salad with Ricotta, 96
Meatballs Hawaiian, 196–97
Mediterranean Strata, 245
Pasta with Fresh Vegetable Sauce,
    220–21
Poached Halibut in Asian Broth,
    118–19
Polenta with Sautéed Vegetables,
    224–25
Pork and Pepper Stew, 210
Ratatouille, 274
Red and Green Pilaf, 264
Roasted Potato and Chicken Salad
    with Greek Dressing, 90–91
Roasted Red Bell Pepper Dip, 31
Seafood Pasta Salad, 88
Slow-Cooker Pepper Steak, 190
Spaghetti with Eggplant Sauce, 227
Spiced Shish Kebabs with
    Horseradish Cream, 186–87
Sweet-and-Sour Broccoli and Red
    Bell Pepper, 251
Triple-Pepper and White Bean
    Soup with Rotini, 69
berries
Blueberry-Yogurt Pancakes, 287
Crepes Suzette with Raspberries,
    312–13
Cumin-Roasted Turkey Breast
    with Raspberry Sauce, 174–75

Maple-Blueberry Bars, 304–5
Very Berry Sorbet, 317
see also cranberries; strawberries
beverages
Orange-Strawberry Froth, 47
Pineapple Shake, 48
Sangría-Style Pomegranate
    Coolers, 46
Spiced Apple Cider, 49
Black-Eyed Pea Salad, Lemon-
    Curried, 84–85
blood cholesterol, 2, 22, 343–45
blood pressure, 2, 347
blueberries
Blueberry-Yogurt Pancakes, 287
Maple-Blueberry Bars, 304–5
body mass index (BMI), 22–23
bok choy
Chinese-Style Chicken and Soba
    Noodles, 160–61
cook's tip on, 219
Soba Lo Mein with Edamame and
    Vegetables, 218–19
bouquet garni, cook's tip on, 49
bran
Cardamom-Lemon Muffins, 281
Pineapple-Carrot Muffins, 284–85
wheat, cook's tip on, 285
breads and breakfast dishes
Blueberry-Yogurt Pancakes, 287
Breakfast Crostini, 290
Breakfast Tortilla Wrap, 291
Cardamom-Lemon Muffins, 281
French Toast with Peach and
    Praline Topping, 292
Oatmeal-Fruit Muffins, 282–83
Pecan-Topped Cinnamon
    Oatmeal, 286
Pineapple-Carrot Muffins, 284–85

breads and breakfast dishes (*cont.*)
    Puffed Pancake with Apple-
        Cranberry Sauce, 288–89
    Speckled Spoon Bread, 280
    Zucchini Bread, 278–79
broccoli
    Broccoli-Cheese Soup, 62
    Skillet Salmon with Broccoli and
        Rice, 124
    Sweet-and-Sour Broccoli and Red
        Bell Pepper, 251
    Thai Chicken with Basil and
        Vegetables, 166–67
    Thai Coconut Curry with
        Vegetables, 238–39
    Triple Vegetable Bake, 272–73
    Vegetable Pancakes, 275
Brussels Sprouts, Roasted, 252
bulgur
    Bulgur and Butternut Squash, 228
    Bulgur and Ground Beef
        Casserole, 191
    Chicken and Veggie Bake, 169
    cook's tip on, 86
    Tabbouleh, 86–87
Burgers, Bunless Beef-and-Bean, 202
buttermilk
    cook's tip on, 121
    Parmesan-Peppercorn Ranch
        Dressing, 100

C

cabbage
    Asian-Style Slaw, 78–79
    Quinoa in Vegetable Nests, 229
    Sautéed Greens and Cabbage, 261
    Stir-Fried Cabbage with Noodles,
        253

    Stuffed Cabbage Rolls, 194–95
    Tilapia Tacos with Roasted-
        Tomato Salsa, 128–29
Cajun seasoning blend, cook's tip on,
    137
cakes
    Banana Mini Snack Cakes, 45
    Chocolate Mini-Cheesecakes, 297
    Lemon Poppy Seed Cake, 294–95
    Pumpkin-Carrot Cake, 296
capers
    Creamy Caper Dip, 30
    Mussels with Yogurt-Caper Sauce,
        134–35
    Tilapia Piccata, 126–27
    Turkey Meatballs in Squash Shells,
        176–77
    Wilted Spinach, 268
Cardamom-Lemon Muffins, 281
carrots
    Apple-Lemon Carrots, 255
    Asian-Style Slaw, 78–79
    Carrot and Barley Pilaf, 254
    Chicken and Vegetable Lasagna,
        170–71
    Chinese-Style Chicken and Soba
        Noodles, 160–61
    Country-Style Vegetable Soup, 55
    Pan-Fried Pasta Pancake with
        Vegetables, 226
    Pineapple-Carrot Muffins, 284–85
    Poached Halibut in Asian Broth,
        118–19
    Pumpkin-Carrot Cake, 296
    Quinoa in Vegetable Nests, 229
    Soba Lo Mein with Edamame and
        Vegetables, 218–19
    Thai Chicken with Basil and
        Vegetables, 166–67

Thai Coconut Curry with
    Vegetables, 238–39
catfish
    Confetti Catfish Fillets, 110
    Crisp Catfish with Creole Sauce,
        112–13
    Crunchy Italian Catfish, 111
cauliflower
    Cauliflower au Gratin, 256–57
    Vegetable Pancakes, 275
cheese
    Breakfast Tortilla Wrap, 291
    Broccoli-Cheese Soup, 62
    Canapés with Roasted Garlic,
        Artichoke, and Chèvre
        Spread, 41
    Cauliflower au Gratin, 256–57
    Chicken and Tortilla Casserole,
        150–51
    Chicken and Vegetable Lasagna,
        170–71
    Chicken Breasts Stuffed with
        Ricotta and Goat Cheese, 146–47
    Chocolate Mini-Cheesecakes, 297
    Country-Style Vegetable Soup, 55
    Eggplant Parmigiana, 234–35
    Fiesta Black Bean Nachos, 232
    Greek Chopped Salad, 93
    Green Bean and Toasted Pecan
        Salad, 76
    Grilled Pizza with Grilled
        Vegetables, 212–13
    Grilled Vegetable Quesadillas,
        230–31
    Macaroni Salad with Ricotta, 96
    Mediterranean Strata, 245
    Parmesan, cook's tip on, 225
    Parmesan-Peppercorn Ranch
        Dressing, 100

Pasta-Parmesan Soup, 57
Pasta with Fresh Vegetable Sauce,
    220–21
Pork with Corn-Cilantro Pesto,
    206–7
Pumpkin Gnocchi, 216–17
Rosemary-Artichoke Frittata,
    240–41
Seafood and Lemon Risotto, 138–39
Spinach and Black Bean
    Enchiladas, 233
Taco Salad, 94–95
Tomato Bursts, 37
Twice-Baked Potatoes and Herbs,
    262
Watercress-Cheese Soufflé, 242–43
Zesty Potato Skins, 42–43
Cheesecakes, Chocolate Mini-, 297
Cherry-Pear Turnovers, 300–1
chicken
    Artichoke-Rotini Salad with
        Chicken, 92
    Asian Grilled Chicken, 142–43
    Brunswick Stew, 163
    Cajun Chicken Pasta, 165
    Chicken and Tortilla Casserole,
        150–51
    Chicken and Vegetable Lasagna,
        170–71
    Chicken and Veggie Bake, 169
    Chicken Breasts Stuffed with
        Ricotta and Goat Cheese,
        146–47
    Chicken Fajitas, 154–55
    Chicken Pot Pie with Mashed
        Potato Topping, 172–73
    Chicken Southwestern, 156–57
    Chicken with Mushroom-Sherry
        Sauce, 152

chicken (*cont.*)

Chicken with Spicy Black Pepper Sauce, 153

Chinese-Style Chicken and Soba Noodles, 160–61

Creamy Chicken Curry, 158–59

Crispy Oven-Fried Chicken, 144

Garlic Chicken Fillets in Balsamic Vinegar, 145

Greek-Style Stewed Chicken, 168

Herbed Chicken Salad, 89

Moroccan Chicken, 164

Orange-Ginger Chicken Skewers, 40

Quick Curry-Baked Chicken with Cucumber Raita, 148–49

Roasted Potato and Chicken Salad with Greek Dressing, 90–91

Slow-Cooker Tuscan Chicken, 162

Spicy Chickpea and Chayote Soup, 68

Thai Chicken with Basil and Vegetables, 166–67

chiles

Bunless Beef-and-Bean Burgers, 202

Chicken and Tortilla Casserole, 150–51

Chicken Southwestern, 156–57

Chili, 200–1

Creamy Chicken Curry, 158–59

Edamame Stir-Fry, 244

handling, cook's tip on, 101

Jícama and Grapefruit Salad with Ancho-Honey Dressing, 80–81

Salmon and Rotini with Chipotle Cream, 125

Seared Tuna with Mango-Pear Salsa, 140

Southwestern Black Bean Spread, 35

Taco Salad, 94–95

Thai Chicken with Basil and Vegetables, 166–67

Tilapia Tacos with Roasted-Tomato Salsa, 128–29

Tomatillo-Avocado Dressing, 101

Chili, 200–1

Chive Dumplings, Tiny, 258

chocolate

Chocolate Soufflés with Vanilla Sauce, 309

Trail Mix with Cocoa-Dusted Almonds, 38

cholesterol, 2, 22, 343–45

Chowder, Hearty Fish, 108–9

Chutney, Nectarine-Plum, 39

Cider, Spiced Apple, 49

cilantro

Bulgur and Ground Beef Casserole, 191

Jícama and Grapefruit Salad with Ancho-Honey Dressing, 80–81

Pork with Corn-Cilantro Pesto, 206–7

Taco Salad, 94–95

citrus

juicing, cook's tip on, 136

zest, cook's tip on, 87

zesting, cook's tip on, 85

see also grapefruit; lemon; limes; orange

coconut

Coconut Cornflake Cookies, 308

Thai Coconut Curry with Vegetables, 238–39

Cod, Grilled, with Artichoke-Horseradish Sauce, 114–15

cookies and bars
 Coconut Cornflake Cookies, 308
 Maple-Blueberry Bars, 304–5
 Nutty Meringue Kisses, 307
cook's tips
 almond flour, 305
 apricot nectar, 47
 asparagus, 59
 avocados, 35
 basmati rice, 265
 beating egg whites, 309
 blending hot liquids, 58
 bok choy, 219
 bouquet garni, 49
 bulgur, 86
 buttermilk, 121
 butternut squash, 267
 chopping fresh herbs, 83
 citrus zest, 87
 coring apples, 298
 corn, 231
 Creole or Cajun seasoning blend,
  137
 curry paste, 239
 cutting dried fruit, 266
 cutting mangoes, 161
 dried fruit, 283
 dried mushrooms, 65
 dry-roasting nuts and seeds in the
  oven, 38
 dry-roasting nuts and seeds on the
  stovetop, 36
 egg whites, 243
 fish sauce, 167
 five-spice powder, 79
 freezing gingerroot, 237
 fresh beets, 249
 fresh mussels, 135
 fresh rosemary, 180

 garam masala, 159
 gingerroot, 183
 grapefruit, 72
 green onions, 147
 handling hot chiles, 101
 hard-boiling eggs, 268
 healthy cuts of steak, 185
 jícama, 81
 juicing citrus, 136
 leftover fresh herbs, 262
 lemons, 87
 measuring sticky foods, 83
 orange-flower water, 73
 panko, 257
 Parmesan cheese, 225
 pears, 301
 peppercorns, 181
 poppy seeds, 295
 quinoa, 229
 rhubarb, 299
 sesame oil, 65
 sesame seeds, 295
 sherry, 109
 skinning poultry, 143
 smoked paprika, 31
 smoked salmon, 32
 storing garlic, 134
 tamari sauce, 109
 Thai basil, 167
 trout, 133
 turmeric, 237
 unprocessed wheat bran, 285
 wheat berries, 63
 white whole-wheat flour, 283
 zesting citrus, 85
corn
 Brunswick Stew, 163
 cook's tip on, 231
 Edamame Stir-Fry, 244

corn (*cont.*)
Grilled Vegetable Quesadillas,
230–31
Individual Corn Puddings, 259
Lemon-Curried Black-Eyed Pea
Salad, 84–85
Pork with Corn-Cilantro Pesto,
206–7
Speckled Spoon Bread, 280
Thai Coconut Curry with
Vegetables, 238–39
Cornflake Coconut Cookies, 308
cornmeal
Polenta with Sautéed Vegetables,
224–25
Speckled Spoon Bread, 280
couscous
Grilled Portobello Mushrooms
with Couscous and Greens,
222–23
Moroccan Chicken, 164
cranberries
Cherry-Pear Turnovers, 300–1
Citrus Rice Salad, 82–83
Grilled Portobello Mushrooms
with Couscous and Greens,
222–23
Pecan-Topped Cinnamon
Oatmeal, 286
Puffed Pancake with Apple-
Cranberry Sauce, 288–89
Creole seasoning blend, cook's tip
on, 137
Crepes Suzette with Raspberries,
312–13
Croquettes, Ham and Rice, 204–5
Crostini, Breakfast, 290
Crust, Gingersnap and Graham
Cracker, 303

cucumbers
Cucumber-Melon Salad with
Raspberry Vinegar, 75
Greek Chopped Salad, 93
Quick Curry-Baked Chicken
with Cucumber Raita,
148–49
Smoked Salmon Dip with
Cucumber and Herbs, 32
Cumin-Roasted Turkey Breast with
Raspberry Sauce, 174–75
curried dishes
Creamy Chicken Curry, 158–59
Lemon-Curried Black-Eyed Pea
Salad, 84–85
Quick Curry-Baked Chicken with
Cucumber Raita, 148–49
Spicy Lentil Curry, 236–37
Thai Coconut Curry with
Vegetables, 238–39
curry paste, cook's tip on, 239

D
dairy products
in healthy diet, 8–9
see also cheese; yogurt
desserts, list of, 293
diabetes, 348
dietary fats, 12–13, 17
dining out strategies, 339–42
dips. *See* appetizers and snacks
dried plums
Skillet Pork Chops with
Cinnamon-Apple Salsa,
209
Sweet-Spice Vanilla Dip with
Dried Plums and Pecans, 33
Dumplings, Tiny Chive, 258

E

edamame
  Edamame Stir-Fry, 244
  Soba Lo Mein with Edamame and
    Vegetables, 218–19
eggplant
  Eggplant Parmigiana, 234–35
  Polenta with Sautéed Vegetables,
    224–25
  Ratatouille, 274
  Spaghetti with Eggplant Sauce,
    227
eggs
  Breakfast Tortilla Wrap, 291
  Chocolate Soufflés with Vanilla
    Sauce, 309
  egg whites, cook's tips on, 243, 309
  hard-boiling, cook's tip on, 268
  Watercress-Cheese Soufflé, 242–43
  Wilted Spinach, 268
egg substitute
  Breakfast Crostini, 290
  Hot-and-Sour Soup with Exotic
    Mushrooms, 64–65
  Mediterranean Strata, 245
  Pasta-Parmesan Soup, 57
  Rosemary-Artichoke Frittata,
    240–41
Enchiladas, Spinach and Black Bean,
  233
exercise, 3, 19–22

F

Fajitas, Chicken, 154–55
fats, dietary, 12–13, 17
Fennel-Orange Salad, 74
fish
  Baked Flounder and Tomatoes, 116
  Broiled Salmon with Olive Pesto,
    122
  Confetti Catfish Fillets, 110
  Crisp Catfish with Creole Sauce,
    112–13
  Crunchy-Crusted Salmon, 120–21
  Crunchy Italian Catfish, 111
  Fish Fillets with Broiled-Veggie
    Rice, 106–7
  Fish Roll-Ups with Spinach, 104–5
  Grilled Cod with Artichoke-
    Horseradish Sauce, 114–15
  Halibut Kebabs, 117
  healthy cooking tips, 330
  in healthy diet, 9–10
  Hearty Fish Chowder, 108–9
  Jamaican Jerk Tuna Steaks, 131
  Mediterranean Grilled Salmon, 123
  Poached Halibut in Asian Broth,
    118–19
  Salmon and Rotini with Chipotle
    Cream, 125
  Seafood Pasta Salad, 88
  Seared Tuna with Mango-Pear
    Salsa, 140
  Skillet Salmon with Broccoli and
    Rice, 124
  smoked salmon, cook's tip on, 32
  Smoked Salmon Dip with
    Cucumber and Herbs, 32
  Tilapia Piccata, 126–27
  Tilapia Tacos with Roasted-
    Tomato Salsa, 128–29
  Tilapia with Lemon-Crumb
    Topping, 130
  trout, cook's tip on, 133
  Trout Amandine with Orange-
    Dijon Sauce, 132–33
  see also shellfish

fish sauce, cook's tip on, 167
five-spice powder, cook's tip on, 79
Flounder and Tomatoes, Baked, 116
flour, white whole-wheat, cook's tip on, 283
French Toast with Peach and Praline Topping, 292
Frittata, Rosemary-Artichoke, 240–41
fruit nectars
    cook's tip on, 47
    Orange-Strawberry Froth, 47
fruits
    Coconut Cornflake Cookies, 308
    dried, cook's tip on, 283
    dried, cutting, cook's tip on, 266
    in healthy diet, 6
    Oatmeal-Fruit Muffins, 282–83
    Praline Butternut Squash, 266–67
    see also berries; *specific fruits*

G

garam masala, cook's tip on, 159
garlic
    Canapés with Roasted Garlic, Artichoke, and Chèvre Spread, 41
    Garlic Chicken Fillets in Balsamic Vinegar, 145
    storing, cook's tip on, 134
Gazpacho Dressing, 99
gingerroot
    Chilled Asparagus Soup, 58–59
    Chinese-Style Chicken and Soba Noodles, 160–61
    Creamy Chicken Curry, 158–59
    Crispy Oven-Fried Chicken, 144
    fresh, cook's tips on, 183, 237
    Fresh Peach and Ginger Crisp, 302

Grilled Teriyaki Sirloin, 182–83
Meatballs Hawaiian, 196–97
Orange-Ginger Chicken Skewers, 40
Poached Halibut in Asian Broth, 118–19
Quick Curry-Baked Chicken with Cucumber Raita, 148–49
Spicy Lentil Curry, 236–37
Sweet-and-Sour Broccoli and Red Bell Pepper, 251
Gingersnap and Graham Cracker Crust, 303
Gnocchi, Pumpkin, 216–17
Graham Cracker and Gingersnap Crust, 303
grains
    bulgur, cook's tip on, 86
    Bulgur and Butternut Squash, 228
    Bulgur and Ground Beef Casserole, 191
    Cardamom-Lemon Muffins, 281
    Carrot and Barley Pilaf, 254
    Chunky Barley Soup, 54
    Creamy Wild Rice and Wheat Berry Soup, 63
    in healthy diet, 7
    Pineapple-Carrot Muffins, 284–85
    Polenta with Sautéed Vegetables, 224–25
    quinoa, cook's tip on, 229
    Quinoa in Vegetable Nests, 229
    Speckled Spoon Bread, 280
    Tabbouleh, 86–87
    wheat berries, cook's tip on, 63
    see also oats; rice
grapefruit
    Boston Citrus Salad, 72–73
    cook's tip on, 72

Jícama and Grapefruit Salad with
Ancho-Honey Dressing, 80–81
green beans
Green Bean and Toasted Pecan
Salad, 76
Pumpkin Gnocchi, 216–17
Roasted Potato and Chicken Salad
with Greek Dressing, 90–91
Salmon and Rotini with Chipotle
Cream, 125
Sweet-Tart Green Beans, 260
green onions, cook's tip on, 147
greens
Fennel-Orange Salad, 74
Grilled Portobello Mushrooms
with Couscous and Greens,
222–23
Gumbo with Greens and Ham,
60–61
Kale-and-Ham-Stuffed Cremini
Mushrooms, 44
Sautéed Greens and Cabbage, 261
Watercress-Cheese Soufflé, 242–43
see also bok choy; cabbage; salads;
spinach
grilled dishes
Asian Grilled Chicken, 142–43
Grilled Cod with Artichoke-
Horseradish Sauce, 114–15
Grilled Pizza with Grilled
Vegetables, 212–13
Grilled Portobello Mushrooms
with Couscous and Greens,
222–23
Grilled Sirloin Steak with
Chimichurri Sauce, 184–85
Grilled Teriyaki Sirloin, 182–83
Grilled Vegetable Quesadillas,
230–31

Jamaican Jerk Tuna Steaks, 131
Mediterranean Grilled Salmon,
123
Gumbo with Greens and Ham,
60–61

H
halibut
Halibut Kebabs, 117
Poached Halibut in Asian Broth,
118–19
ham
Gumbo with Greens and Ham,
60–61
Ham and Rice Croquettes,
204–5
Kale-and-Ham-Stuffed Cremini
Mushrooms, 44
HDL cholesterol, 22, 344
healthy cooking strategies
baking, 330
braising, 325–26
broiling, 327
cooking tips, 330–32
grilling, 326
microwaving, 327
poaching, 328
roasting, 329
steaming, 328
stewing, 326
stir-frying, 329
healthy lifestyle
committing to, 3
drinking in moderation, 24
managing your weight, 21–23
physical activity, 19–22
quitting smoking, 24
regular doctor visits, 24

heart disease
  heart attack warning signs, 349–50
  reducing risk of, 2–3
  risk factors, 1–2, 346–48
  stroke warning signs, 350
heart-healthy diet
  added sugars, 14–16
  basic nutrition guidelines, 5–6
  dairy products, 8–9
  dining out strategies, 339–42
  effect on cholesterol, 2–3
  fats and oils, 12–13
  fish and seafood, 9–10
  fruits and vegetables, 6
  grains, 7–8
  healthy shopping strategies, 319–24
  heart-healthy pantry staples, 333–38
  portion control, 16–17
  poultry and meat, 10–11
  sodium, 14
herbs
  Creamy Herb Dressing, 98
  fresh, cook's tips on, 83, 262
  Smoked Salmon Dip with Cucumber and Herbs, 32
  Twice-Baked Potatoes and Herbs, 262
  see also specific herbs
honey, measuring, cook's tip on, 83
horseradish
  Beef Tenderloin Roast, 180–81
  Crisp Catfish with Creole Sauce, 112–13
  Grilled Cod with Artichoke-Horseradish Sauce, 114–15
  Spiced Shish Kebabs with Horseradish Cream, 186–87
hot liquids, blending, cook's tip on, 58

I

Ice, Strawberry Margarita, 318

J

jícama
  cook's tip on, 81
  Jícama and Grapefruit Salad with Ancho-Honey Dressing, 80–81
  Taco Salad, 94–95

K

Kale-and-Ham-Stuffed Cremini Mushrooms, 44

L

Lasagna, Chicken and Vegetable, 170–71
LDL cholesterol, 22, 344
legumes
  Lemon-Curried Black-Eyed Pea Salad, 84–85
  Spicy Lentil Curry, 236–37
  see also beans
lemon
  Apple-Lemon Carrots, 255
  Cardamom-Lemon Muffins, 281
  Citrus-Tarragon Vinaigrette, 102
  cook's tip on, 87
  Lemon-Curried Black-Eyed Pea Salad, 84–85
  Lemon Poppy Seed Cake, 294–95
  Light and Lemony Spinach Soup, 52
  Seafood and Lemon Risotto, 138–39
  Tabbouleh, 86–87
  Tilapia Piccata, 126–27

Tilapia with Lemon-Crumb
Topping, 130
Lentil Curry, Spicy, 236–37
limes
Sangría-Style Pomegranate
Coolers, 46
Strawberry Margarita Ice, 318

M
mango
Chinese-Style Chicken and Soba
Noodles, 160–61
cutting, cook's tip on, 161
Mango Brûlée with Pine Nuts, 310
Seared Tuna with Mango-Pear
Salsa, 140
Summertime Soup, 56
Maple-Blueberry Bars, 304–5
meat
healthy cooking tips, 330–31
in healthy diet, 10–11
see also beef; pork
meatballs
Meatballs Hawaiian, 196–97
Turkey Meatballs in Squash Shells,
176–77
Meat Loaf with Apricot Glaze, 192–93
melon
Cucumber-Melon Salad with
Raspberry Vinegar, 75
Summertime Soup, 56
Meringue Kisses, Nutty, 307
molasses, measuring, cook's tip
on, 83
muffins
Cardamom-Lemon Muffins, 281
Oatmeal-Fruit Muffins, 282–83
Pineapple-Carrot Muffins, 284–85

mushrooms
Balsamic Braised Beef with Exotic
Mushrooms, 188
Breakfast Crostini, 290
Chicken and Veggie Bake, 169
Chicken with Mushroom-Sherry
Sauce, 152
Chinese-Style Chicken and Soba
Noodles, 160–61
dried, cook's tip on, 65
Grilled Pizza with Grilled
Vegetables, 212–13
Grilled Portobello Mushrooms with
Couscous and Greens, 222–23
Hearty Fish Chowder, 108–9
Hot-and-Sour Soup with Exotic
Mushrooms, 64–65
Kale-and-Ham-Stuffed Cremini
Mushrooms, 44
Pasta with Fresh Vegetable Sauce,
220–21
Rosemary-Artichoke Frittata,
240–41
Sirloin Steak with Portobello
Mushrooms, 189
Triple Vegetable Bake, 272–73
Turkey Patties with Fresh Basil-
Mushroom Sauce, 178
Vegetable Pancakes, 275
Warm Mushroom Salad, 77
mussels
fresh, cook's tip on, 135
Mussels with Yogurt-Caper Sauce,
134–35

N
Nachos, Fiesta Black Bean, 232
Nectarine-Plum Chutney, 39

noodles
    Cajun Red Scallops, 136–37
    Chinese-Style Chicken and Soba
        Noodles, 160–61
    Soba Lo Mein with Edamame and
        Vegetables, 218–19
    Stir-Fried Cabbage with Noodles,
        253
nutrition facts panels, 319–22
nutrition guidelines, 5–6
nuts
    dry-roasting, cook's tips on, 36, 38
    see also almonds; pecans; pine nuts;
        walnuts

O

oats
    Apple-Rhubarb Crisp, 298–99
    Crunchy-Crusted Salmon, 120–21
    Fresh Peach and Ginger Crisp, 302
    Maple-Blueberry Bars, 304–5
    Oatmeal-Fruit Muffins, 282–83
    Pecan-Topped Cinnamon
        Oatmeal, 286
obesity, 347–48
oils, 12–13, 17
okra
    Gumbo with Greens and Ham,
        60–61
    Red and Green Pilaf, 264
olives
    Broiled Salmon with Olive Pesto, 122
    Fresh Basil and Kalamata
        Hummus, 34
    Greek Chopped Salad, 93
    Greek-Style Stewed Chicken, 168
    Macaroni Salad with Ricotta, 96
    Moroccan Chicken, 164

    Roasted Potato and Chicken Salad
        with Greek Dressing, 90–91
    Slow-Cooker Tuscan Chicken, 162
    Tomato Bursts, 37
    Zesty Potato Skins, 42–43
onions
    Chicken Fajitas, 154–55
    Chicken Pot Pie with Mashed
        Potato Topping, 172–73
    green, cook's tip on, 147
    Halibut Kebabs, 117
    Poached Halibut in Asian Broth,
        118–19
    Ratatouille, 274
    Soba Lo Mein with Edamame and
        Vegetables, 218–19
    Spiced Shish Kebabs with
        Horseradish Cream, 186–87
    Thai Chicken with Basil and
        Vegetables, 166–67
orange
    Beets in Orange Sauce, 248–49
    Boston Citrus Salad, 72–73
    Citrus Rice Salad, 82–83
    Crepes Suzette with Raspberries,
        312–13
    Fennel-Orange Salad, 74
    Herbed Chicken Salad, 89
    Orange-Ginger Chicken
        Skewers, 40
    Orange-Strawberry Froth, 47
    Sangría-Style Pomegranate
        Coolers, 46
    Strawberry Margarita Ice, 318
    Trout Amandine with Orange-
        Dijon Sauce, 132–33
orange-flower water
    Boston Citrus Salad, 72–73
    cook's tip on, 73

P

pancakes
  Blueberry-Yogurt Pancakes, 287
  Pan-Fried Pasta Pancake with
    Vegetables, 226
  Puffed Pancake with Apple-
    Cranberry Sauce, 288–89
  Vegetable Pancakes, 275
panko, cook's tip on, 257
parsley
  Grilled Sirloin Steak with
    Chimichurri Sauce, 184–85
  Tabbouleh, 86–87
pasta
  Artichoke-Rotini Salad with
    Chicken, 92
  Cajun Chicken Pasta, 165
  Chicken and Vegetable Lasagna,
    170–71
  Macaroni Salad with Ricotta, 96
  Pan-Fried Pasta Pancake with
    Vegetables, 226
  Pasta e Fagioli, 214–15
  Pasta-Parmesan Soup, 57
  Pasta with Fresh Vegetable Sauce,
    220–21
  Pumpkin Gnocchi, 216–17
  Rustic Tomato Soup, 66–67
  Salmon and Rotini with Chipotle
    Cream, 125
  Seafood Pasta Salad, 88
  Spaghetti with Eggplant Sauce, 227
  Triple-Pepper and White Bean
    Soup with Rotini, 69
  see also couscous; noodles
peaches
  Bananas Foster Plus, 315
  French Toast with Peach and
    Praline Topping, 292

  Fresh Peach and Ginger Crisp,
    302
  Honey-Baked Pecan Peaches, 311
  Summertime Soup, 56
pears
  Cherry-Pear Turnovers, 300–1
  cook's tip on, 301
  Seared Tuna with Mango-Pear
    Salsa, 140
pecans
  French Toast with Peach and
    Praline Topping, 292
  Fresh Peach and Ginger Crisp,
    302
  Green Bean and Toasted Pecan
    Salad, 76
  Honey-Baked Pecan Peaches, 311
  Mock Baklava, 306
  Nutty Meringue Kisses, 307
  Pecan-Topped Cinnamon
    Oatmeal, 286
  Praline Butternut Squash, 266–67
  Quinoa in Vegetable Nests, 229
  Sweet-Spice Vanilla Dip with
    Dried Plums and Pecans, 33
peppercorns
  cook's tip on, 181
  Parmesan-Peppercorn Ranch
    Dressing, 100
peppers. See bell peppers; chiles
pesto
  Broiled Salmon with Olive Pesto,
    122
  Pork with Corn-Cilantro Pesto,
    206–7
phyllo dough
  Cherry-Pear Turnovers, 300–1
  Mock Baklava, 306
physical activity, 3, 19–22

physical inactivity, 347
pineapple
    Jamaican Jerk Tuna Steaks, 131
    Meatballs Hawaiian, 196–97
    Pineapple-Carrot Muffins, 284–85
    Pineapple Shake, 48
    Praline Butternut Squash, 266–67
    Zucchini Bread, 278–79
pine nuts
    Asparagus with Dill and Pine
        Nuts, 250
    Broiled Salmon with Olive Pesto,
        122
    Mango Brûlée with Pine Nuts, 310
Pizza, Grilled, with Grilled
    Vegetables, 212–13
Plum-Nectarine Chutney, 39
Polenta with Sautéed Vegetables,
    224–25
Pomegranate Coolers,
    Sangía-Style, 46
poppy seeds
    Banana Mini Snack Cakes, 45
    cook's tips on, 295
    Lemon Poppy Seed Cake, 294–95
    Oven-Fried Green Tomatoes with
        Poppy Seeds, 269
pork
    Breakfast Tortilla Wrap, 291
    Hot-and-Sour Soup with Exotic
        Mushrooms, 64–65
    Pork and Pepper Stew, 210
    Pork with Corn-Cilantro Pesto,
        206–7
    Pork with Savory Sauce, 203
    Skillet Pork Chops with
        Cinnamon-Apple Salsa, 209
    Spicy Baked Pork Chops, 208
    see also ham

portion control, 16–17
potatoes
    Breakfast Tortilla Wrap, 291
    Chicken Pot Pie with Mashed
        Potato Topping, 172–73
    Country-Style Vegetable Soup, 55
    Hearty Fish Chowder, 108–9
    Roasted Potato and Chicken Salad
        with Greek Dressing, 90–91
    Sweet Potatoes in Creamy
        Cinnamon Sauce, 263
    Triple Vegetable Bake, 272–73
    Twice-Baked Potatoes and Herbs,
        262
    Zesty Potato Skins, 42–43
Pot Pie, Chicken, with Mashed Potato
    Topping, 172–73
poultry
    healthy cooking tips, 330–31
    in healthy diet, 10–11
    skinning, cook's tip on, 143
    see also chicken; turkey
Puddings, Individual Corn, 259
pumpkin
    Pumpkin-Carrot Cake, 296
    Pumpkin Gnocchi, 216–17

Q

Quesadillas, Grilled Vegetable, 230–31
quinoa
    cook's tip on, 229
    Quinoa in Vegetable Nests, 229

R

raisins
    Apple-Raisin Sauce, 314
    Mock Baklava, 306

Trail Mix with Cocoa-Dusted
Almonds, 38
Zucchini Bread, 278–79
raspberries
Crepes Suzette with Raspberries,
312–13
Cumin-Roasted Turkey Breast
with Raspberry Sauce, 174–75
Ratatouille, 274
recipes
adapting favorite recipes, 332–33
healthy cooking strategies, 325–32
ingredient equivalents, 323–24
nutritional analyses, 27–28
stocking heart-healthy pantry, 333–38
rhubarb
Apple-Rhubarb Crisp, 298–99
cook's tip on, 299
rice
basmati, cook's tip on, 265
Citrus Rice Salad, 82–83
Creamy Wild Rice and Wheat
Berry Soup, 63
Fish Fillets with Broiled-Veggie
Rice, 106–7
Golden Rice, 265
Gumbo with Greens and Ham, 60–61
Ham and Rice Croquettes, 204–5
Jamaican Jerk Tuna Steaks, 131
Meatballs Hawaiian, 196–97
Red and Green Pilaf, 264
Seafood and Lemon Risotto, 138–39
Skillet Salmon with Broccoli and
Rice, 124
Slow-Cooker Pepper Steak, 190
Stuffed Cabbage Rolls, 194–95
Thai Chicken with Basil and
Vegetables, 166–67
Risotto, Seafood and Lemon, 138–39

rosemary
fresh, cook's tip on, 180
Rosemary-Artichoke Frittata,
240–41

S
salad dressings
Citrus-Tarragon Vinaigrette, 102
Creamy Artichoke Dressing, 97
Creamy Herb Dressing, 98
Gazpacho Dressing, 99
Parmesan-Peppercorn Ranch
Dressing, 100
Tomatillo-Avocado Dressing, 101
salads
Artichoke-Rotini Salad with
Chicken, 92
Asian-Style Slaw, 78–79
Boston Citrus Salad, 72–73
Citrus Rice Salad, 82–83
Cucumber-Melon Salad with
Raspberry Vinegar, 75
Fennel-Orange Salad, 74
Greek Chopped Salad, 93
Green Bean and Toasted Pecan
Salad, 76
Herbed Chicken Salad, 89
Jícama and Grapefruit Salad with
Ancho-Honey Dressing, 80–81
Lemon-Curried Black-Eyed Pea
Salad, 84–85
Macaroni Salad with Ricotta, 96
Roasted Potato and Chicken Salad
with Greek Dressing, 90–91
Seafood Pasta Salad, 88
Tabbouleh, 86–87
Taco Salad, 94–95
Warm Mushroom Salad, 77

salmon
  Broiled Salmon with Olive Pesto, 122
  Crunchy-Crusted Salmon, 120–21
  Mediterranean Grilled Salmon, 123
  Salmon and Rotini with Chipotle Cream, 125
  Skillet Salmon with Broccoli and Rice, 124
  smoked, cook's tip on, 32
  Smoked Salmon Dip with Cucumber and Herbs, 32
salsa
  Seared Tuna with Mango-Pear Salsa, 140
  Skillet Pork Chops with Cinnamon-Apple Salsa, 209
  Tilapia Tacos with Roasted-Tomato Salsa, 128–29
sauces
  Apple-Raisin Sauce, 314
  healthy cooking tips, 331
scallops
  Cajun Red Scallops, 136–37
  Seafood and Lemon Risotto, 138–39
seeds
  dry-roasting, cook's tips on, 36, 38
  Trail Mix with Cocoa-Dusted Almonds, 38
  see also poppy seeds; sesame seeds
serving sizes, 16–17
sesame oil, cook's tip on, 65
sesame seeds
  cook's tips on, 295
  Grilled Teriyaki Sirloin, 182–83
shellfish
  Cajun Red Scallops, 136–37
  healthy cooking tips, 330
  in healthy diet, 9–10

mussels, cook's tip on, 135
Mussels with Yogurt-Caper Sauce, 134–35
Seafood and Lemon Risotto, 138–39
sherry
  Chicken with Mushroom-Sherry Sauce, 152
  cook's tip on, 109
  Hearty Fish Chowder, 108–9
side dishes, list of, 247
Slaw, Asian-Style, 78–79
slow-cooker dishes
  Chinese-Style Chicken and Soba Noodles, 160–61
  Slow-Cooker Pepper Steak, 190
  Slow-Cooker Tuscan Chicken, 162
smoked paprika, cook's tip on, 31
smoking, 24, 348
snow peas
  Hot-and-Sour Soup with Exotic Mushrooms, 64–65
  Pan-Fried Pasta Pancake with Vegetables, 226
  Seafood and Lemon Risotto, 138–39
sodium, 14
Sorbet, Very Berry, 317
soufflés
  Chocolate Soufflés with Vanilla Sauce, 309
  Watercress-Cheese Soufflé, 242–43
soups
  Broccoli-Cheese Soup, 62
  Chilled Asparagus Soup, 58–59
  Chunky Barley Soup, 54
  Country-Style Vegetable Soup, 55
  Creamy Wild Rice and Wheat Berry Soup, 63
  Gumbo with Greens and Ham, 60–61

healthy cooking tips, 331
Hearty Fish Chowder, 108–9
Hot-and-Sour Soup with Exotic
    Mushrooms, 64–65
Light and Lemony Spinach
    Soup, 52
Pasta-Parmesan Soup, 57
Rustic Tomato Soup, 66–67
Silky Winter-Squash Soup, 53
Spicy Chickpea and Chayote
    Soup, 68
Summertime Soup, 56
Triple-Pepper and White Bean
    Soup with Rotini, 69
see also stews
spinach
    Chicken and Vegetable Lasagna,
        170–71
    Fish Roll-Ups with Spinach,
        104–5
    Greek Chopped Salad, 93
    Light and Lemony Spinach
        Soup, 52
    Spinach and Black Bean
        Enchiladas, 233
    Wilted Spinach, 268
Spoon Bread, Speckled, 280
spreads. *See* appetizers and snacks
squash
    Bulgur and Butternut Squash, 228
    butternut, cook's tip on, 267
    Edamame Stir-Fry, 244
    Fish Fillets with Broiled-Veggie
        Rice, 106–7
    Grilled Vegetable Quesadillas,
        230–31
    Polenta with Sautéed Vegetables,
        224–25
    Praline Butternut Squash, 266–67

Silky Winter-Squash Soup, 53
Spicy Chickpea and Chayote
    Soup, 68
Turkey Meatballs in Squash Shells,
    176–77
see also pumpkin; zucchini
stews
    Brunswick Stew, 163
    Chili, 200–1
    Pork and Pepper Stew, 210
    Ratatouille, 274
sticky foods, measuring, cook's tip
    on, 83
Strata, Mediterranean, 245
strawberries
    Orange-Strawberry Froth, 47
    Strawberries Romanoff, 316
    Strawberry Margarita Ice, 318
    Summertime Soup, 56
stroke warning signs, 350
sugars, added, 14–16
sugar snap peas
    Grilled Teriyaki Sirloin, 182–83
    Soba Lo Mein with Edamame and
        Vegetables, 218–19
Sweet Potatoes in Creamy Cinnamon
    Sauce, 263

T

Tabbouleh, 86–87
tacos
    Southwestern Beef Pita Tacos,
        198–99
    Tilapia Tacos with Roasted-
        Tomato Salsa, 128–29
Taco Salad, 94–95
tamari sauce, cook's tip on, 109
Tarragon-Citrus Vinaigrette, 102

tilapia
  Tilapia Piccata, 126–27
  Tilapia Tacos with Roasted-
    Tomato Salsa, 128–29
  Tilapia with Lemon-Crumb
    Topping, 130
tofu
  Eggplant Parmigiana, 234–35
  Thai Coconut Curry with
    Vegetables, 238–39
tomatillos
  Chicken and Tortilla Casserole,
    150–51
  Tomatillo-Avocado Dressing, 101
tomatoes
  Baked Flounder and Tomatoes, 116
  Brunswick Stew, 163
  Bulgur and Ground Beef
    Casserole, 191
  Chicken Southwestern, 156–57
  Greek Chopped Salad, 93
  Greek-Style Stewed Chicken, 168
  Mediterranean Grilled Salmon,
    123
  Mediterranean Strata, 245
  Oven-Fried Green Tomatoes with
    Poppy Seeds, 269
  Pasta with Fresh Vegetable Sauce,
    220–21
  Ratatouille, 274
  Rosemary-Artichoke Frittata,
    240–41
  Rustic Tomato Soup, 66–67
  Skillet Salmon with Broccoli and
    Rice, 124
  Slow-Cooker Pepper Steak, 190
  Slow-Cooker Tuscan Chicken, 162
  Spaghetti with Eggplant Sauce,
    227

  Spiced Shish Kebabs with
    Horseradish Cream, 186–87
  Stovetop Scalloped Tomatoes,
    270
  Stuffed Zucchini, 271
  Tabbouleh, 86–87
  Taco Salad, 94–95
  Tilapia Tacos with Roasted-
    Tomato Salsa, 128–29
  Tomato Bursts, 37
  Triple-Pepper and White Bean
    Soup with Rotini, 69
tortillas
  Breakfast Tortilla Wrap, 291
  Chicken and Tortilla Casserole,
    150–51
  Chicken Fajitas, 154–55
  Grilled Vegetable Quesadillas,
    230–31
  Spinach and Black Bean
    Enchiladas, 233
  Tilapia Tacos with Roasted-
    Tomato Salsa, 128–29
Trail Mix with Cocoa-Dusted
  Almonds, 38
triglycerides, 345
trout
  cook's tip on, 133
  Trout Amandine with Orange-
    Dijon Sauce, 132–33
tuna
  Jamaican Jerk Tuna Steaks, 131
  Seafood Pasta Salad, 88
  Seared Tuna with Mango-Pear
    Salsa, 140
turkey
  Cumin-Roasted Turkey Breast
    with Raspberry Sauce,
    174–75

Turkey Meatballs in Squash Shells, 176–77
Turkey Patties with Fresh Basil-Mushroom Sauce, 178
turmeric, cook's tip on, 237

V

vegetables
Chicken and Vegetable Lasagna, 170–71
Chicken Pot Pie with Mashed Potato Topping, 172–73
Country-Style Vegetable Soup, 55
Grilled Pizza with Grilled Vegetables, 212–13
Grilled Vegetable Quesadillas, 230–31
healthy cooking tips, 331
in healthy diet, 6
Pan-Fried Pasta Pancake with Vegetables, 226
Pasta with Fresh Vegetable Sauce, 220–21
Polenta with Sautéed Vegetables, 224–25
Quinoa in Vegetable Nests, 229
Soba Lo Mein with Edamame and Vegetables, 218–19
Thai Coconut Curry with Vegetables, 238–39
Triple Vegetable Bake, 272–73
Vegetable Pancakes, 275
see also specific vegetables
vegetarian entrées
Bulgur and Butternut Squash, 228
Edamame Stir-Fry, 244

Eggplant Parmigiana, 234–35
Fiesta Black Bean Nachos, 232
Grilled Pizza with Grilled Vegetables, 212–13
Grilled Portobello Mushrooms with Couscous and Greens, 222–23
Grilled Vegetable Quesadillas, 230–31
Macaroni Salad with Ricotta, 96
Mediterranean Strata, 245
Pan-Fried Pasta Pancake with Vegetables, 226
Pasta e Fagioli, 214–15
Pasta with Fresh Vegetable Sauce, 220–21
Polenta with Sautéed Vegetables, 224–25
Pumpkin Gnocchi, 216–17
Quinoa in Vegetable Nests, 229
Rosemary-Artichoke Frittata, 240–41
Rustic Tomato Soup, 66–67
Soba Lo Mein with Edamame and Vegetables, 218–19
Spaghetti with Eggplant Sauce, 227
Spicy Chickpea and Chayote Soup, 68
Spicy Lentil Curry, 236–37
Spinach and Black Bean Enchiladas, 233
Thai Coconut Curry with Vegetables, 238–39
Triple-Pepper and White Bean Soup with Rotini, 69
Watercress-Cheese Soufflé, 242–43
Vinaigrette, Citrus-Tarragon, 102

W

walnuts
Mock Baklava, 306
Nutty Meringue Kisses, 307
Pumpkin-Carrot Cake, 296
Trail Mix with Cocoa-Dusted
Almonds, 38
Zucchini Bread, 278–79
Zucchini Spread, 36
water chestnuts
Chicken and Veggie Bake, 169
Chinese-Style Chicken and Soba
Noodles, 160–61
Hot-and-Sour Soup with Exotic
Mushrooms, 64–65
watercress
Gumbo with Greens and Ham,
60–61
Watercress-Cheese Soufflé,
242–43
weight, healthy, 21
weight, unhealthy, 347–48
wheat berries
cook's tip on, 63
Creamy Wild Rice and Wheat
Berry Soup, 63
wheat bran
Pineapple-Carrot Muffins, 284–85
unprocessed, cook's tip on, 285
white whole-wheat flour, cook's tip
on, 283
Wild Rice and Wheat Berry Soup,
Creamy, 63

Y

yogurt
Blueberry-Yogurt Pancakes, 287
Creamy Caper Dip, 30
Creamy Herb Dressing, 98
Mussels with Yogurt-Caper Sauce,
134–35
Quick Curry-Baked Chicken with
Cucumber Raita, 148–49
Strawberries Romanoff, 316
Sweet-Spice Vanilla Dip with
Dried Plums and Pecans, 33
Trout Amandine with Orange-
Dijon Sauce, 132–33

Z

zucchini
Chicken and Vegetable Lasagna,
170–71
Country-Style Vegetable Soup, 55
Grilled Pizza with Grilled
Vegetables, 212–13
Ham and Rice Croquettes, 204–5
Mediterranean Strata, 245
Polenta with Sautéed Vegetables,
224–25
Ratatouille, 274
Stuffed Zucchini, 271
Triple-Pepper and White Bean
Soup with Rotini, 69
Zucchini Bread, 278–79
Zucchini Spread, 36